A Comprehensive Guide to Radiographic Sciences and Technology

A Comprehensive Guide to Radiographic Sciences and Technology

Euclid Seeram, PhD, MSc, BSc, FCAMRT

Full Member – Health Physics Society

ACADEMIC APPOINTMENTS
Adjunct Associate Professor; Medical Imaging and Radiation Sciences; Monash University, Melbourne, Australia I Adjunct Professor; Faculty of Science; Charles Sturt University, Bathurst, Australia I Adjunct Professor; Medical Radiation Sciences, Faculty of Health; University of Canberra, Canberra, Australia

WILEY Blackwell

Registered Office(s)
John Wiley & Sons, Inc., 111 River Street, Hoboken, NJ 07030, USA
John Wiley & Sons Ltd, The Atrium, Southern Gate, Chichester, West Sussex, PO19 8SQ, UK

Editorial Office
9600 Garsington Road, Oxford, OX4 2DQ, UK

For details of our global editorial offices, customer services, and more information about Wiley products visit us at www.wiley.com.

Wiley also publishes its books in a variety of electronic formats and by print-on-demand. Some content that appears in standard print versions of this book may not be available in other formats.

Library of Congress Cataloging-in-Publication Data

Names: Seeram, Euclid, author.
Title: A comprehensive guide to radiographic sciences and technology / Euclid Seeram.
Description: First edition. | Hoboken, NJ : Wiley-Blackwell, 2021. | Includes bibliographical references and index.
Identifiers: LCCN 2020050277 (print) | LCCN 2020050278 (ebook) | ISBN 9781119581840 (paperback) | ISBN 9781119581833 (adobe pdf) | ISBN 9781119581857 (epub)
Subjects: MESH: Radiography–methods | Radiography–instrumentation | Image Processing, Computer-Assisted | Technology, Radiologic | Radiation Protection
Classification: LCC RC78.2 (print) | LCC RC78.2 (ebook) | NLM WN 200 | DDC 616.07/572–dc23
LC record available at https://lccn.loc.gov/2020050277
LC ebook record available at https://lccn.loc.gov/2020050278

Cover Design: Wiley
Cover Image: © Cybrain/iStock/Getty Images

Set in 10/12pt Trade Gothic by SPi Global, Pondicherry, India

Printed in Singapore
M097082_260321

Dedication

This book is dedicated with love to my Family; my lovely wife, Trish; our son David and
daughter-in-law Priscilla; and our two very smart, cute,
and witty granddaughters, Claire and Charlotte

Contents

SECTION 1: INTRODUCTION

SECTION 2: BASIC RADIOGRAPHIC SCIENCES AND TECHNOLOGY

SECTION 3: COMPUTED TOMOGRAPHY: BASIC PHYSICS AND TECHNOLOGY

SECTION 4: CONTINUOUS QUALITY IMPROVEMENT

Foreword

Dr Euclid Seeram is a recognized educator in the field of radiographic sciences, including computed tomography (CT) physics and instrumentation for radiologic technologists/radiographers. He has published over 22 textbooks on various topics related to these two subjects. His textbooks can be found in universities and colleges around the world that offer medical imaging and radiographic science programs. He has a very well-developed approach in all his textbooks that allows the reader to understand complex topics.

Dr Seeram has decades of experience in the teaching radiographic sciences and CT. Euclid is also a highly regarded researcher in this field, gaining a PhD in digital radiography and radiation dose management strategies. He has continued to work and research in this area. Euclid is also a highly sought-after speaker and provides highly engaging talks and presentations on radiographic sciences and CT. The impact of Euclid's texts, journal articles, and presentations has had on radiologic technologists/radiographers, other related individuals, and medical physicists in their understanding of radiographic sciences and CT, cannot be understated.

The development of the technologies that underpin radiological science continues to grow rapidly and at an increasing rate. Students need to understand these technologies and the implications of these technologies in clinical practice. The approach undertaken by Dr Seeram in this text, *A Comprehensive Guide to Radiographic Sciences and Technology*, is to provide readers with clearly defined chapters on several related topics. The chapters and sections of this book are logically structured so the readers/learners can progress their understanding. Of growing importance in radiographic sciences, and often misunderstood, is the understanding of the radiation dose/image quality relationship of digital radiography. This area has a strong focus in this textbook. Furthermore, the knowledge gained from studying the subject matter covered in this book will benefit technologists/radiographers in clinical practice in order to provide tangible benefits to their patients.

I have been fortunate to know Dr Seeram for over 20 years, initially as his PhD supervisor, and now as a coresearcher, colleague, and friend/mate. Euclid continues to amaze me on his dedication and passion to educate radiologic technologists/radiographers and his drive to continue writing. Euclid must be commended for his continued efforts in making radiographic sciences, and CT knowledge easy to understand by students and practitioners.

Dr Robert Davidson, PhD, MAppSc (MI), BBus, FASMIRT
Professor of Medical Imaging, Faculty of Health,
University of Canberra, ACT, Australia

Preface

Radiographic sciences and technology include a wide range of topics essential for radiography/radiological technology curriculum offered by educational institutions (colleges, universities, and institutes of technology) around the world. Additionally, radiography/radiological technology/medical imaging professional organizations for radiographer/technologist education and training, such as, for example, the American Association of Radiologic Technologists (ASRT) and the Canadian Association of Medical Radiation Technologists (CAMRT) offer curriculum guidelines for educational institutions to use as guiding principles for core clinical competencies. More details of related activities are highlighted in Chapter 1.

This book includes 13 chapters organized into 6 sections as follows:

- *Section 1*: Chapters 1 and 2
- *Section 2*: Basic Radiographic Sciences and Technology
- *Section 3*: Computed Tomography: Basic Physics and Technology
- *Section 4:* Continuous Quality Improvement
- *Section 5*: Picture Archiving and Communications Systems (PACS) and Imaging Informatics
- *Section 6:* Radiation Protection

PURPOSE

The purpose of this book, *A Comprehensive Guide to Radiographic Sciences and Technology*, is to provide an essential and practical guide for students and technologists engaged in the study and practice of radiography/radiological technology. One of its primary goals is to provide a resource that is brief, clear, and a concise coverage of the subject in preparation for final examinations as well as professional certification examinations. This book is not a textbook as such, and it is not intended to replace the vast resources on radiographic sciences and technology. Rather, it provides a précis of the extensive coverage of radiographic sciences and technical system components for students and technologists.

A Comprehensive Guide to Radiographic Sciences and Technology · Preface

xv

CORE OBJECTIVES

On the successful completion of the chapters in this book, the reader will be able to:

1. Outline the core subject matter content of radiographic imaging modalities.
2. Identify and describe briefly the major technical components of digital radiographic imaging systems.
3. Outline the basic physics necessary for understanding essential concepts and principles for x-ray generation, production, x-ray emission, x-ray interaction with matter, and radiation attenuation in the production of diagnostic images in clinical practice.
4. Describe the major components of the x-ray generator and x-ray tube including heat capacity and heat dissipation and x-ray beam filtration and collimation.
5. Explain the core principles of digital image processing, including the characteristics of the digital image and common image processing operations applied in practice.
6. Identify and explain the fundamental physics principles and technology of the following digital imaging modalities: computed radiography (CR), flat-panel digital radiography (FPDR), and digital fluoroscopy.
7. Identify image quality metrics and explain each of them with a focus on how dose is linked to image quality.
8. Describe the basic physics of computed tomography (CT) and explain the major technological considerations of multislice CT (MSCT), including image post processing, image quality metrics, and radiation protection considerations in CT.
9. Identify the essential elements of quality control (QC), including the principles of a repeat analysis, and describe the performance criteria for common QC tests for radiography, fluoroscopy, and CT.
10. Describe the core technical components of PACS, and explain briefly the general subject matter comprising imaging informatics, including artificial intelligence and its subsets: machine learning and deep learning.
11. Outline the major principles of radiobiology, with a specific focus on relevant physical processes, dose–response models, stochastic and deterministic effects, as well as radiation effects on the conceptus.
12. Explain the technical factors affecting the dose in radiography, fluoroscopy, and CT.
13. Identify and discuss the major components of radiation protection including radiation protection philosophy of the International Commission on Radiological Protection (ICRP), radiation quantities and units, personnel dosimetry, optimization of radiation protection, and the current state of gonadal shielding.

USE OF THESE OBJECTIVES AND CONTENT

These objectives and content covered in this book may be used in the following subjects covered in standard radiography/radiological technology programs:

1. Physics of Radiography
2. Digital Radiography Equipment Including Digital Fluoroscopy
3. Image Quality
4. PACS and Imaging Informatics
5. Quality Control in Radiography and Fluoroscopy

6. Computed Tomography Physics and Instrumentation for Entry to Practice
7. Radiobiology for Diagnostic Radiography
8. Radiation Protection in Diagnostic Radiography

Chapter 1 introduces the nature and scope of radiographic sciences and technology and sets the general framework for the remaining chapters. Whereas Chapter 2 presents a description of the major technical components of digital radiographic imaging modalities, such as computed radiography (CR), FPDR, digital fluoroscopy, and digital mammography, Chapter 3 describes the essential physics of radiography, including principles for x-ray generation, production, x-ray emission, x-ray interaction with matter, and radiation attenuation in the production of diagnostic images in clinical practice. Chapter 4 examines the major technical components of the x-ray generator and x-ray tube, describing core technologies such as the x-ray circuit, x-ray generators, the structure and function of the x-ray tube, heat capacity and dissipation, as well as the nature of x-ray beam filtration and collimation. Chapter 5 reviews the fundamental elements of digital image processing beginning with a definition, followed by a review of image formation and representation, processing operations, characteristics of digital images, and gray-scale processing, most notably the nature of windowing. Chapters 6 and 7 address the principles and technology of digital radiographic imaging modalities, identified in Chapter 2, and image quality and dose, respectively. Chapter 8 covers the essential technical aspects of CT, at a depth needed for entry-to-practice, including the basic physics and technology of CT. Specifically, the major technical system components of MSCT are described. Furthermore, image processing, image quality, and radiation dose and radiation protection are described. Chapter 9 provides a discussion of quality control and focusses on the performance criteria/tolerance limits for common QC tests for radiography, fluoroscopy, and CT tests that are in the domain of the technologist. Finally, the chapter reviews the elements of repeat image analysis. The nature of imaging informatics including major topics as picture archiving and communication systems (PACS), and specific imaging topics such as enterprise imaging, cloud computing, Big Data, and artificial intelligence, and its subsets, machine learning and deep learning, are reviewed in Chapter 10. Finally, Section 6 covers topics in radiation protection. In particular, while Chapter 11 provides a discussion of basic concepts of radiobiology, Chapter 12 deals with the technical dose factors in radiography, fluoroscopy, and CT. Finally, the book concludes with Chapter 13, which addresses the essential principles of radiation protection, focusing on topics such as a rationale for radiation protection, objectives of radiation protection, radiation protection philosophy of the International Commission on Radiological Protection (ICRP), radiation quantities and units, personnel dosimetry, optimization of radiation protection, and the current state of gonadal shielding.

Enjoy the pages that follow and remember – your patients will benefit from your wisdom.

Euclid Seeram, PhD., MSc., BSc., FCAMRT
British Columbia, Canada

Acknowledgments

It is always a pleasure to acknowledge the contributions of experts in the field of radiographic sciences including radiologic physics, equipment, image quality, quality control, radiobiology and radiation protection from whom I have learned a great deal that allows me to write this book.

First, I am indeed grateful to all those who have dedicated their energies in providing several comprehensive volumes on radiologic physics and instrumentation for the radiologic community. I would like to acknowledge the notable medical physicist, Dr. Stewart Bushong ScD, FAAPM, FACR and experimental radiobiologist, Dr. Elizabeth Travis, PhD. I have learned a great deal on radiologic science from the works of Dr. Bushong, a professor of radiologic science in the Department of Radiology, Baylor College of Medicine, Houston, TX. In addition, I have gained further insight into the nature, scope, and depth of radiobiology and particularly its significance in radiology, from Dr. Travis, a researcher in the Department of Experimental Radiotherapy, University of Texas, MD Anderson Cancer Center, Houston, TX.

Secondly, I am grateful to physicist, Dr. Hans Swan, PhD and digital radiography expert, Dr. Rob Davidson, PhD, who served as my primary supervisors for my PhD dissertation entitled *Optimization of the Exposure Indicator of a Computed Radiography Imaging System as a Radiation Dose Management Strategy*. Furthermore, Dr. Stewart Bushong served as an external examiner for my PhD dissertation. Additionally, two other notable medical physicists from whom I have learned my digital radiography imaging physics and technology are Dr. Charles Willis, PhD (University of Texas; MD Anderson Cancer Center-Retired) and Dr. Anthony Seibert, PhD (University of California at Davis). Dr. Seibert's notable textbook on *The Essential Physics of Medical Imaging* has educated me in the core principles of medical imaging physics. Thanks to you all.

I must acknowledge all others, such as the authors whose papers I have cited and referenced in this book, thank you for your significant contributions to radiographic sciences knowledge base. Additionally, I would like to express my sincere thanks to Dr. Perry Sprawls, PhD, FACR, FAAPM, FIOMP, Distinguished Emeritus Professor, Emory University, Director, Sprawls Educational Foundation, http://www.sprawls.org, Co-Director, College on Medical Physics, ICTP, Trieste, Italy, and Co-Editor, Medical Physics International, http://www.mpijournal.org/.

Dr. Sprawls has always supported my writing and I appreciate his free resources on the World Wide Web (www) from which students, technologists, and educators alike can benefit. I must also mention Dr. Anthony Wolbarst, PhD, Medical Physics Department, University of Kentucky (Retired).

Another individual to whom I owe a good deal of thanks is Valentina Al Hamouche, MRT(R), MSc, who is the CEO/Founder VCA Education Solutions for Health Professionals http://www.VCAeducation.ca. Valentina has provided me with opportunities to provide radiographic sciences and CT physics and Instrumentation in-house lectures and webinars to further educate technologists and students across Canada and internationally. Thanks Valentina.

I must acknowledge James Watson, Commissioning Editor, Wiley, Oxford, UK, who understood and evaluated the need for this book. Additionally, I am grateful to Anupama Sreekanth, former project editor and current managing editor Anne Hunt at Wiley, for the advice and support you both provided to me during the writing stage of this book. Furthermore, I appreciate the work of Sandeep Kumar, Content Refinement Specialist at Wiley, who has done an excellent job in bringing this manuscript to fruition.

Finally, I am very grateful for the warm and wonderful support of my family: my lovely wife, Trish, a very wise and caring person; and my very smart son, David, a very special young man and the best Dad in the universe. Thank you both for your unending love, support, and encouragement.

Last, but not least, I want to express my gratitude to all the students in my radiographic sciences classes – your questions have provided me with a further insight into teaching this important subject. Thank you.

SECTION 1

Introduction

1

Radiographic sciences and technology: an overview

Radiographic Science and Technology have evolved through the years, ever since the discovery and use of x-rays in 1895. This evolution has resulted in the introduction of physical principles and technology with the major goal of improving the care and management of the patient. Furthermore, a significant benefit of these innovations is focused on reducing the radiation dose to the patient without compromising image quality. *Radiographic sciences* deal with the physics of various diagnostic imaging modalities (radiography, fluoroscopy, mammography, and computed tomography [CT]) and include x-ray generation, x-ray production, x-ray emission, and x-ray interaction with tissues. Furthermore, radiographic sciences also address radiation risks and radiation protection. *Radiographic technology,* on the other hand, addresses the equipment components and how they function to produce diagnostic images, image quality characteristics, and quality control (QC) aspects of these imaging modalities.

A Comprehensive Guide to Radiographic Sciences and Technology, First Edition. Euclid Seeram.
© 2021 John Wiley & Sons Ltd. Published 2021 by John Wiley & Sons Ltd.

The workhorse of radiology has been *film-screen radiography* which is now obsolete and has been replaced globally with *digital imaging*. The scope of digital imaging is extremely wide and now involves a basic understanding of computer sciences, to explain how the new digital imaging modalities work. These modalities include computed radiography (CR), flat-panel digital radiography (FPDR), digital fluoroscopy (DF), digital mammography (DM), digital tomosynthesis, and CT. In addition, the digital imaging environment now demands that operators understand what has been referred to as "imaging informatics," an area of study that involves picture archiving and communication systems (PACS), enterprise imaging, Big Data, machine learning (ML), deep learning (DL), and artificial intelligence (AI).

With the above in mind, various professional organizations such as the American Society of Radiologic Technologists (ASRT), the Canadian Association of Medical Radiation Technologists (CAMRT), and other professional medical imaging organizations throughout the world have prescribed curricula for diagnostic imaging programs which provide guiding, principles that assist academic program leaders in designing foundational learning outcomes that are intended to meet the professional standards, and more importantly meet the entry requirements for clinical practice. Institutions offering educational programs in diagnostic imaging should be then able to raise the level of these foundational learning outcomes and content to meet the requirements of degree programs, including graduate degree programs in diagnostic imaging.

A good example of the above is offered by the ASRT curriculum content which is organized around the following subject matter [1]: Introduction to Radiologic Science and Health Care; Ethics and Law in the Radiologic Sciences; Human Anatomy and Physiology; Pharmacology and Venipuncture; Imaging Equipment; Radiation Production and Characteristics; Principles of Exposure and Image Production; Digital Image Acquisition and Display; Image Analysis; Radiation Biology; Radiation Protection; Clinical Practice; Patient Care in Radiologic Sciences; Radiographic Procedures; Radiographic Pathology; Additional Modalities and Radiation Therapy; Basic Principles of Computed Tomography and Sectional Anatomy. Similar content is characteristic of other curricula offered by other medical imaging professional organizations around the world.

Keeping the above ideas in mind, this book will address content that are considered radiographic sciences and technology. Specifically, the chapters included present a summary of the critical knowledge base needed for effective and efficient imaging of the patient, and wise use of the technical factors that play a significant role in optimization of the dose to the patient without compromising the image quality necessary for diagnostic interpretation. Furthermore, the summaries of the technical elements of radiographic sciences and technology will assist the student in preparing to write certification examinations. As such, the major and significant principles and concepts will be reviewed in three sections as follows:

Section 1: Radiographic imaging systems: major modalities and components
Section 2: Radiographic physics and technology
Section 3: Radiation protection and dose optimization

RADIOGRAPHIC IMAGING SYSTEMS: MAJOR MODALITIES AND COMPONENTS

In this book, the following *radiographic imaging systems* will be reviewed. These include x-ray imaging modalities such as digital radiography (DR) which includes CR and FPDR, DF, DM, digital radiographic and breast tomosynthesis, and CT. Furthermore, these systems include imaging informatics which has become commonplace since radiology and more importantly hospitals are now all operating in the digital environment; that is, all data acquired from the patient are now in digital form and are stored and communicated using digital technologies. Informatics topics of importance include that nature and scope of PACS, enterprise imaging, cloud computing, Big Data, and the more recent of computer applications in medical imaging: AI. More details of these major technologies and how they work will be presented in Chapter 6 on Digital Imaging Modalities and Chapter 10 on Imaging Informatics.

RADIOGRAPHIC PHYSICS AND TECHNOLOGY

Radiographic physics and technology subject matter include basic physics concepts, and more specifically the physics of diagnostic imaging; technical aspects of the modalities; radiographic exposure technique; image quality, quality assurance (QA), and QC; CT physical principles; imaging informatics; radiobiology and radiation protection.

Essential physics of diagnostic imaging

The *physics of diagnostic imaging* is an important and vital topic that explains the nature of how these imaging modalities work to produce diagnostic images of the patient. Understanding the fundamental physics will provide the user with the tools not only needed to produce optimum image quality but more importantly to protect the patient from unnecessary radiation. As such, it is now a common characteristic of imaging departments to optimize radiation dose and work within the International Commission on Radiological Protection (ICRP) philosophy of as low as reasonably achievable (ALARA) to reduce the dose to the patient but not compromise the diagnostic quality of the images used to make a diagnosis of the patient's medical condition.

In this book, the topics in physics that will emphasize the imaging modalities are the nature of radiation, x-ray generation, x-ray production, x-ray emission, x-ray attenuation, and x-ray interaction with matter. Furthermore, other physics topics of significance are radiation quantities and their associated units and measurement concepts. These topics and more fall in the domain of *Health Physics*. Three radiation quantities that are important to radiation protection of the patient are exposure, absorbed dose, and effective dose (ED). The units associated with each of these include coulombs per kilogram (C/kg), Grays (Gy), and Sieverts (Sv), respectively. In order to measure radiation, it must first be detected.

Digital radiographic imaging modalities

As listed earlier in this chapter, these modalities include CR, FPDR or DR as it is sometimes referred to, DF, DM, digital radiographic tomosynthesis (DRT), digital breast tomosynthesis (DBT), and last but not least CT. Additionally, since all of the above-mentioned modalities include image processing using computers, the concepts of Digital Image Processing will be reviewed since it has become an essential tool for technologists, radiologists, and medical physicists working in a digital radiology department.

These imaging modalities include specific physics concepts that must be understood for optimum results. For example, CR is based on the use of photostimulable phosphors (PSP) which are based on the physical principle of photostimulable luminescence (PSL). An example of one such phosphor is barium fluoro halide (BaFX) where the halide (X) can be chlorine (Cl), bromine (Br), iodine (I), or a mixture of them. When the PSP imaging plate (IP) is exposed to x-rays, electrons are moved from the ground state (valence band) to a higher energy level (conducting band) and are trapped there until the PSP plate is exposed to a laser light and subsequently the electrons in the higher energy state return to their ground state, thus emitting a bluish-purple light referred to as PSL.

The detectors used in FPDR are based on semiconductor physics. Examples of two such common detectors used in DR are indirect digital detectors which use amorphous silicon photoconductor coupled to an x-ray scintillator (cesium iodide for example) and direct digital detectors which use amorphous selenium photoconductor. While the former detector converts x-rays to light which falls upon the silicon photoconductor to produce electrical signals, the latter detector converts x-rays directly into electrical signals. The other digital imaging modality detectors are based on photoconductor physics.

The imaging modalities listed above convert radiation attenuated by the patient and falling on the digital detector to digital data. This is necessary since computers are used to process these data through popular digital image processing operations. These operations have become commonplace and must be fully understood for effective use in clinical practice. One such tool is the concept of windowing, where the image brightness and contrast can be changed by the operator to suit the viewing needs of the human interpreter. Furthermore, other digital image processing tools that are vital in DBT and CT image reconstruction algorithms. These algorithms have evolved from the filtered back projection (FBP) algorithm to more complex algorithms such as iterative reconstruction (IR) algorithms. These algorithms play an important role in building up an image from data collected through 360° around the patient in CT, for example. Today, IR algorithms are now used by all CT vendors.

Radiographic exposure technique

Radiographic exposure technique refers to the use of exposure factors coupled with other elements on the x-ray control panel, selected by the technologist to produce diagnostic images. Exposure factors include the kilovoltage (kV), the milliamperes (mA), and exposure time (s) and the selection of the appropriate source-to-image receptor distance (SID). Furthermore, the proper positioning of the patient and image receptor, tube alignment with the image receptor, use of appropriate filtration and collimation, and patient instructions, are all the other elements that play an important role during the radiographic examination.

Image quality considerations

Image quality is a significant goal of radiographic imaging modalities. The attenuated radiation data from the patient are used to create images that are used for diagnostic interpretation by a human observer. There are at least five important descriptors of digital image quality and these include spatial resolution, contrast resolution, noise, detective quantum efficiency (DQE), and image artifacts. While spatial resolution addresses the sharpness of images, and is related to the size of the pixels (picture elements) in an image, contrast resolution or density resolution deals with the ability of the imaging system to demonstrate differences in tissue contra, and is linked to the bit depth, that is the range of gray levels per pixel. Noise, on the other hand, depends on the number of x-ray photons used to create the image. While fewer photons (low exposure technique factors) will result in more noise (grainy appearance), more photons (higher exposure technique factors) will create a better image (less noisy image), but at the expense of dose. Another digital image quality descriptor is the DQE, which is a measure of the efficiency and fidelity with which the detector can convert an input exposure into a useful output image. Finally, digital images are not free of artifacts. These are features seen on the image that are not present in the patient, and can pose challenges for the human observer in detecting fact from artifact.

Computed tomography – physics and instrumentation

This section will present a broad overview of the essential elements of the *Physics and Instrumentation of Computed Tomography*. One of the major advantages of CT is that it provides improved contrast resolution compared to radiography and for this reason, it has proven to be worthy of further developments in imaging soft tissues of the human body. It is important to note, however, that magnetic resonance imaging (MRI) has superior contrast resolution compared to all other imaging modalities, such as radiography, nuclear medicine, and diagnostic medical sonography.

CT is a sectional imaging technique that produces direct cross-sectional digital images referred to as transverse axial images which has been referred to as planar sections that are perpendicular to the long axis of the patient. The word "computed" implies that a computer is used to process and reconstruct x-ray transmission data collected from the patient. The CT scanner has evolved from single-slice CT scanners (SSCT) to multi-slice CT scanners (MSCT). State-of-the-art CT scanners are now MSCT scanners capable of a wide range of applications. The increasing use is that CT in clinical practice has led to increasing doses to the patient and a well-documented fact is that CT delivered the highest collective dose in the United States compared to other medical imaging modalities.

Two individuals shared the Nobel Prize in Medicine and Physiology in 1979 for their development of the CT scanner. These include Godfrey Newbold Hounsfield in the United Kingdom (UK) who invented the first clinically useful scanner, and Allan Cormack, a physicist at Tufts University in Massachusetts.

CT is a multidisciplinary technology and has its roots in physics, mathematics, engineering, and computer science. The CT process consists of at least three major system components that are used to produce the CT image; the data acquisition system; the computer system; and the image display, storage, and communication systems.

Data acquisition means that radiation attenuation data are collected from the patient during the scanning. In this respect, an x-ray tube coupled to special electronic detectors rotate around the patient to collect and measure attenuation readings as the x-ray beam passes through the patient.

The attenuation is according to Beer–Lambert's law:

$$I = I_0 e^{-\mu \Delta x},$$

where I is the transmitted x-ray beam intensity, I_0 is the original x-ray beam intensity, e represents Euler's constant, μ is the linear attenuation coefficient, and Δx is the finite thickness of the section. In CT, the system calculates all μs for all structures seen on the image. Special detectors and detector electronics are used to calculate the attenuation data and convert them into integers (0, a positive number, or a negative number) referred to as CT numbers using an image reconstruction algorithm to build up the image in numerical format. The CT numbers (numerical image format) are converted into a gray-scale image for display on a monitor for the observer to interpret.

The CT numbers are calculated using the following relationship:

$$CT\ number = \frac{\mu_{tissue} - \mu_{water}}{\mu_{water}} \cdot K,$$

where K represents a scaling factor. In general, K is equal to 1000. When Hounsfield invented the scanner, K was equal to 500.

The technology aspects of CT are complex and are responsible for using the attenuation values collected around the patient for 360° to build up an image of the internal anatomy of the patient, and displays such image for interpretation by radiologists. The technology addressing the collection of these values includes the x-ray tube which is coupled to special electronic detectors and detector electronics. Another major technology component in CT is the computer system which captures the raw data from the detectors and uses sophisticated image reconstruction algorithms for creating the image from the raw data.

Present-day CT scanners are MSCT scanners. One characteristic feature of MSCT is the two-dimensional detector array, compared to a one-dimensional detector array of SSCT. This means that there will be additional specific technical factors that affect the dose in CT. One such notable factor is the pitch (P), which is defined by the International Electrotechnical Commission (IEC) as the distance the table travels per rotation (D) divided by the total collimation (W). This can be expressed algebraically as:

$$P = D\ /\ W$$

The increasing use of CT has led to widespread concerns about high patient radiation doses from CT examinations relative to other radiography examinations. The distribution of the dose to the patient in CT is significantly different than the distribution of the dose in radiography. These differences require additional CT-specific dose metrics. There are essential four CT-specific dose metrics: the computed tomography dose index (CTDI), the dose length product (DLP), the size-specific dose estimate (SSDE), and the ED. These and other elements of CT physical principles will be described further in Chapter 7.

Quality control

QC is an essential activity of all medical imaging departments and it is part of a QA program. QA deals with people and includes the administrative aspects of patient care and quality outcomes. QC addresses the technical aspects of equipment performance used to image patients. QA and QC programs have evolved into what is now referred to as *Continuous Quality Improvement* (CQI) which includes *Total Quality Management* (TQM). CQI was introduced by the Joint Committee on Accreditation of Healthcare organizations (JCAHO) to stress the importance that all employees play an active role in ensuring a quality product. The purpose of the procedures and techniques of CQI, QA, and QC is threefold: to ensure optimum image quality for the purpose of enhancing diagnosis, to optimize the radiation dose to patients and reduce the dose to personnel, and to reduce costs to the healthcare facility.

An effective QC program consists of at least three major steps, namely acceptance testing, routine performance, and error correction. While acceptance testing is the first major step in a QC program and it ensures that the equipment meets the specifications set by the manufacturers, routine performance involves performing the actual QC test on the equipment with varying degrees of frequencies (annually, semi-annually, monthly, weekly, or daily). Error correction means that equipment not meeting the performance criteria or tolerance limit established for specific QC tests must be replaced or repaired to meet tolerance limits. These limits include both qualitative and quantitative criteria used to assess image quality. For example, the tolerance for collimation of the x-ray beam should be ±2% of the SID.

QC for DR has evolved from simple to more complex tests and test tools to assure that the DR equipment is working properly to meet optimum image quality standards and fall within the ALARA philosophy in radiation protection. The American Association of Physicists in Medicine (AAPM) has recommended that several testing procedures for CR QC, using specific tools developed for CR QC. A few examples of these test procedures include physical inspection of IP, dark noise and uniformity, exposure indicator (EI) calibration, laser beam function, spatial accuracy, erasure thoroughness, aliasing/grid response, positioning and collimation errors, to mention a few.

QC is now an essential requirement of CT imaging and requires that users have a clear understanding of the various tests that play a significant role in dose-image quality optimization.

Imaging informatics at a glance

Imaging Informatics is the current term used by the Society of Imaging Informatics in Medicine (SIIM) to replace the old term medical imaging informatics. SIIM notes that imaging informatics "is the study and application of processes of information and communications technology for the acquisition, manipulation, analysis, and distribution of image data."

Imaging informatics is based on core topics that range from information and communication technologies, PACS, radiology information systems (RIS), the electronic health record, to cloud computing, Big Data, AI, ML, and DL. In this section, these core elements that characterize these topics will only be highlighted as a basis for setting the stage for the more detailed coverage later in the book.

Information technology (IT) refers to the use of computers and computer communications technologies to not only to process, store, secure electronic data but to communicate these data using computer networking infrastructure. PACS is an excellent example of an informatics-rich medical device. PACS include the imaging image acquisition modalities such as digital radiographic and CT modalities, a computer network database server, storage and archival systems, and display workstations. PACS may be connected to information systems such as the RIS and the hospital information system (HIS). Furthermore, these systems must be fully integrated and secured for efficient and effective data interchange. One such approach within the PACS infrastructure is cloud computing, which simply provides a means of using the Internet for storage and retrieval (for example) of data using specific software packages. Additionally, emerging topics which will have an impact on the practice of medical imaging include Big Data, AI, ML, and DL.

Big Data is characterized by four Vs: Volume, Variety, Velocity, and Veracity. While Volume refers to the very large amount of data, Variety deals with a wide array of data from multiple sources. Furthermore, Velocity addresses the very high speeds at which the data are generated. Finally, Veracity describes the uncertainty of the data such as the authenticity and credibility. AI uses computers in an "effort to automate intellectual tasks normally performed by humans." A subset of AI is ML which includes "a set of methods that automatically detect patterns in data, and then utilize the uncovered patterns to predict future data or enable decision making under uncertain conditions." A subset of ML is DL which uses algorithms that are "characterized by the use of neural networks with many layers." These emerging technologies will evolve and more importantly become useful tools in medical imaging. Therefore, students and technologists alike should make every effort to grasp their meaning and applications so that they can communicate effectively with radiologists and medical physics in an effort to participate actively in the management of patient care.

RADIATION PROTECTION AND DOSE OPTIMIZATION

Current radiation protection standards and recommendations for the safe use of ionizing radiation to image humans are based on the fact that exposure to radiation can cause biological effects. These bioeffects fall in the subject matter domain of radiobiology.

Radiobiology

Radiobiology is the study of effects of radiation on biologic systems which occur at the molecular, cellular levels and subsequently leading to whole-body biological effects generally categorized as early and late effects.

The study of radiobiology is vital for technologists and radiologists working in radiology departments, and it involves an understanding of related physics and chemistry, types of biological effects, radiosensitivity, target theory, and direct and indirect effects. Furthermore, radiobiology involves discussing of deterministic effects (early effects) and stochastic effects (late effects). These topics and their associated subtopics (for example, subtopics for stochastic effects are radiation-induced malignancy, and hereditary effects) will be outlined in Chapter 9.

Topics in physics that are significant to radiobiology include atomic structure, the nature and properties of x-rays, ionization, excitation, linear energy transfer (LET), and relative biologic effectiveness (RBE). Additionally, the essential chemistry of the interactions of radiation and patient which occur with water (since the body contains 70–85% water) is the radiolysis of water. Such chemical interactions result in ionization of water, forming ion pairs and free radicals of which the latter can react further to form other molecules that are toxic to the cell.

Two significant and important topics in radiobiology are stochastic and deterministic effects. Stochastic effects are those for which the probability of the effect increases as the dose increases and for which there is no threshold dose. For stochastic effects, there is no risk-free dose. These effects can occur at the local tissue level and can cause life-span shortening, radiation-induced malignancy, and hereditary effects (late effects that occur in the offspring of the irradiated individual). Stochastic effects are classified as late effects, since they occur years after the exposure of the individual. Deterministic effects on the other hand are those effects for which the severity of the effect depends on the dose. These effects have a threshold dose and increase with increasing dose. These effects are called early effects since they can occur within minutes, hours, days, weeks, and months after the exposure.

Radiation protection in diagnostic radiography

The overall objectives of radiation protection are to prevent deterministic effects and minimize the probability of stochastic effects. The current standards for radiation protection of patients in medicine are established by authoritative radiation protection organizations responsible for providing guidelines and recommendations on radiation protection. While some of these address radiation risks, others are devoted to radiation protection based on the radiation risks data. Three such organizations are the International Commission on Radiologic Protection (ICRP), the National Council on Radiation Protection and Measurements (NCRP), and the Food and Drug Administration (FDA), the latter two are in the United States.

Radiation protection criteria and standards are guided by two triads, namely radiation protection principles and radiation protection actions. While the former deals with the ICRP's principles of justification, optimization, and dose limitation, the latter addresses the triad of time, shielding, and distance. The principle of justification is intended for physicians ordering x-ray examinations; it addresses the notion that there should be a net benefit associated with each and every exposure a patient receives. Optimization implies that radiation workers should work within the ALARA philosophy; that is, to obtain the best possible image with the lowest radiation dose and not compromise the image quality. Finally, the dose limits principle deals with the legal limits on the radiation dose received per year or accumulated over a working life-time for persons who are occupationally exposed and for others as well, such as students in training and members of the public.

The triad of radiation protection actions include time, shielding, and distance. To be effective, it is necessary to keep the time of exposure to radiation as short as possible, since the relationship between time and exposure is proportional; that is, if the time of exposure doubles, the exposure doubles. Shielding ensures protection of patients and workers and members of the public through the use of lead shields and aprons for patients and workers, respectively. Furthermore, the walls of x-ray rooms are also shielded using concrete or lead, for example, to prevent exposure of members of the public who are in a waiting room, waiting for patients having x-rays. Finally, exposure is inversely proportional to the distance; that is, the further away individuals are from the source of the radiation, the less exposure they will receive.

The notion of dose limits is vital to radiation protection of occupationally exposed individuals such as technologists, for example, and non-occupationally exposed individuals (members of the public). Essentially, these limits are established by organizations such as the ICRP, and national organizations, to minimize the risks of the stochastic effects of radiation. The ICRP recommended dose limit for occupational exposure, for example, is 20 mSv/year averaged over defined periods of five years.

The *diagnostic reference level* (DRL) is a concept used to address the limits of exposure for patients. DRLs are not equivalent to dose limit s for occupationally and non-occupationally exposed individuals. The DRL has been defined by various radiation protection organizations. One such definition is that of the American College of Radiology (ACR) as "an investigation level to identify unusually high radiation dose or exposure levels for common diagnostic medical x-ray procedures." DRLs are tools that radiology departments can use to measure and assess radiation doses to patients for a defined set of procedures. If the doses delivered are consistently greater than established DRLs for that facility's country or region, then the department should be concerned about its radiation protection procedures, investigate why exposures are beyond the established DRLs, and take corrective action.

Technical factors affecting dose in radiographic imaging

Radiographic imaging includes modalities such as DR, DF, and CT. There are several technical factors including operator-selectable (under the control of the technologist and/or radiologist) factors that affect the dose to the patient and operator. The major factors affecting dose to the patient in DR include beam energy and filtration, exposure technique factors, beam collimation, the size of the x-ray field, the size of the patient, SID, grids, image receptor sensitivity or speed, and DQE. Major technical factors affecting the dose to the patient in fluoroscopy include beam energy or filtration, x-ray tube current, beam-on time, automatic dose-rate control, collimation, source-to-skin distance, patient-to-image intensifier distance, patient size, anti-scatter grids, image magnification, last image hold, image recording method, and pulsed fluoroscopy.

In CT, there are numerous technical factors affecting the dose to patients. Major factors include exposure technique factors, pitch, effective mAs, collimation and slices, overbeaming and over-ranging, automatic tube current modulation, automatic voltage selection, and IR algorithms.

Radiation protection regulations

Radiation protection regulations and guidelines address equipment specifications, procedures for minimizing the dose to patients and personnel, and shielding, outlined in various reports, and are issued by major agencies in respective countries. In the United States (US), for example, while the NCRP deals with medical x-ray, electron beam, and gamma ray protection for energies up to 50 MeV in NCRP Report No. 102: Equipment Design and Use; the Code of Federal Regulations (CFR) Title 21 (US Department of Health and Human Services, Food and Drug Administration [FDA]) deals with the Performance Standards for Ionizing Radiation Emitting Products.

Equipment specifications for radiography, fluoroscopy, and CT are intended for manufacturers. Specifications for radiographic equipment relate to the x-ray control panel, leakage radiation from the x-ray tube, filtration, collimation, SID, source-to-skin distance, and the exposure switch for fixed and mobile radiographic systems. An example of one such recommendation for the exposure switch is that for fixed radiographic equipment, the exposure switch must be on the control panel to ensure that the operator remains in the control booth during the exposure. Furthermore, the switch must be a "dead man" switch; that is, pressure must be applied to the switch for the exposure to occur.

For fluoroscopy, these specifications include specifications for filtration, collimation, source-to-skin distance, exposure switch, cumulative timer, protective curtain, table and Bucky-slot shielding, and accessory protective clothing. The recommendation for protective aprons worn during fluoroscopy is that they shall have at least a 0.5 mm lead equivalent.

Guidelines and regulations also focus on practices and procedures for reducing the dose to patients and personnel and to keep exposures according to the ALARA philosophy. Technologists must refer to the safety codes of their respective countries for more detailed information. Two such examples of these guidelines on radiography and fluoroscopy state that selection and use of the best possible exposure technique factors should keep the dose ALARA without compromising image quality. Additionally, high-kVp techniques reduce the dose to the patient.

Procedural factors for minimizing dose to personnel are wide and varied and technologists must work within the ALARA philosophy to accomplish this task. Two such examples of recommendations to ensure personnel dose reduction are that (i) only essential personnel must be present in an x-ray room during the exposure and (ii) technologists must remain in the control booth during radiographic exposures and must wear protective aprons when the situation makes this impossible. Another significant recommendation relates to shielding, a radiation protection action and design criterion that is intended to protect patients, personnel, and members of the public. Shielding includes specific area shielding (protecting radiosensitive organs) and protective barriers (walls) positioned between the source of radiation and the individual. This type of shielding, for example, is specifically intended to protect personnel and members of the public from unnecessary radiation.

Optimization of radiation protection

The ICRP optimization framework refers to optimization as keeping the dose ALARA and not compromise the diagnostic quality of the image. Therefore, optimization includes image quality and radiation dose.

The journal *Radiation Protection Dosimetry* dedicated a special issue to optimization strategies in medical imaging for fluoroscopy, radiography, mammography, and CT. Several studies identified at least four important requirements for dose and image-quality optimization research. First, patient safety must be a priority in any study. Second, the level of image quality needed for a particular diagnostic task must be determined. The third requirement involves acquiring images at various exposure levels from high to low and in such a manner that accurate diagnosis can still be made, and finally, use reliable and valid methodologies for the dosimetry, image acquisition, and evaluation of image quality using human observers, keeping in mind the nature of the detection task.

An interesting study utilizing these elements of dose optimization is one by Seeram and colleagues published in *Radiologic Technology* in 2016. The purpose was to investigate a technique for optimizing radiation dose and image quality for a CR system. The researchers measure the entrance skin doses for phantom models of the pelvis and lumbar spine imaged using the vendor's recommended exposure settings (i.e. the reference doses) as well as doses above and below the vendor's recommended settings for both body parts. Images were assessed using visual grading analysis (VGA). The phantom dosimetry results revealed strong positive linear relationships between dose and milliampere seconds (mAs), mAs and inverse EI, and dose and inverse EI for both body parts. The VGA showed that optimized values of 16 mAs/EI = 136 for the anteroposterior (AP) pelvis and 32 mAs/EI = 139 for the AP lumbar spine did not compromise image quality. Selecting optimized mAs reduced dose by 36% compared with the vendor's recommended mAs (dose) values. The study concluded that optimizing the mAs and associated EIs can be an ED management strategy.

Bibliography

1. American Society of Radiologic Technologists (2016). *Radiography Curriculum*. Albuquerque, NM: American Society of Radiologic Technologists.
2. Bushong, S. (2017). *Radiologic Science for Technologists*. St Louis, MO: Elsevier.
3. Bushberg, J.T., Seibert, J.A., Leidholdt, E.M. Jr., and Boone, J.M. (2012). *The Essential Physics of Medical Imaging*, 3e. Philadelphia, PA: Wolters Kluwer/Lippincott Williams & Wilkins.
4. Seeram, E. and Brennan, P. (2017). *Radiation Protection in Diagnostic X-Ray Imaging*. Burlington, MA: Jones and Bartlett Learning.
5. Seeram, E. (2016). *Computed Tomography: Physical Principles, Clinical Applications, and Quality Control*. St Louis, MO: Elsevier.
6. Wolbarst, A.B., Capasso, P., and Wyant, A. (2013). *Medical Imaging: Essentials for Physicians*. Hoboken, NJ: Wiley.
7. Seeram, E. (2020). *Rad Tech's Guide to Radiation Protection*, 2e. Hoboken, NJ: Wiley.
8. Seeram, E. (2019). *Digital Radiography: Physical Principles and Quality Control*. Singapore: Springer.

2

Digital radiographic imaging systems: major components

The purpose of this chapter is to present a general overview of the digital radiographic imaging systems used in diagnostic radiology, by describing briefly, the general system components of each of the modalities in an effort to lay the foundations needed for a good understanding of how each component works to create images and protect not only patients but technologists as well. The more technical details will be reviewed in later chapters on each of the modalities. First, it is important to review the essential principles of film-screen radiography (FSR) in order to fully understand the rationale for the emergence of digital imaging modalities.

FILM-SCREEN RADIOGRAPHY: A SHORT REVIEW OF PRINCIPLES

The overall system components of FSR are shown in Figure 2.1. These include the x-ray generator, the x-ray tube, a radiographic table, the image receptor, a chemical processing unit, and a light view-box. A film-based image is created as follows:

A Comprehensive Guide to Radiographic Sciences and Technology, First Edition. Euclid Seeram.
© 2021 John Wiley & Sons Ltd. Published 2021 by John Wiley & Sons Ltd.

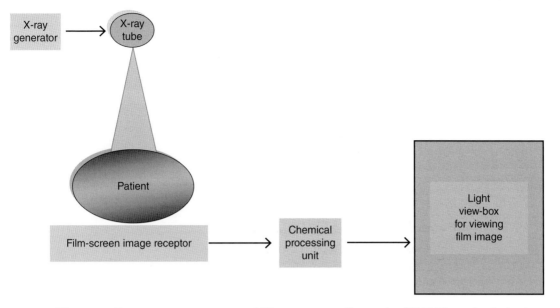

Figure 2.1 The overall system components of film screen radiography (FSR). These include the x-ray generator, the x-ray tube, the image receptor, a chemical processing unit, and a light view-box, for viewing the film image.

1. X-rays pass through the patient and fall upon the film to form a latent image.
2. The latent image is then rendered visible using *chemical processing*.
3. The visible image on the film is displayed on a light view-box for viewing and interpretation by a radiologist. This image consists of varying degrees of blackening as a result of the amount of exposure transmitted by different parts of the anatomy. While the blackening is referred to as the film density, the difference in densities in the image is referred to as the film contrast. The film converts the radiation transmitted through the various types of tissues (tissue contrast) into film contrast.
4. The light from the view-box is transmitted through the film and can be measured using a densitometer and is referred to as the *optical density* (OD), which is defined as the log of the ratio of the intensity of the view-box (original intensity) to the intensity of the transmitted light. The OD is used to describe the degree of film blackening as a result of radiation exposure.
5. A plot of the OD as a function of the log of the relative radiation exposure is described by the well-known characteristic curve (Hurter–Driffield Curve), which provides information about the film response to the exposure (Figure 2.2). There are three parts of the curve: the toe region, the slope, and the shoulder region. Exposures that fall in the toe and shoulder region of the curve will result in images that are light (underexposed) and images that are dark (overexposed), respectively. Acceptable image contrast is obtained when the exposure that falls within the slope of the curve. This slope defines the exposure latitude as well as the film contrast characteristics (the steeper the gradient, the higher the contrast).
6. The density of the image is hence used as an exposure indicator that provides immediate feedback to the technologist that the correct exposure technique factors have been used for the examination. This curve also shows that FSR has a fixed film speed (sensitivity) and a fixed-dose requirement.
7. Furthermore, the characteristic curve can be used to describe the film speed, average gradient, the film gamma, and the film latitude. Only film speed and film latitude will be reviewed

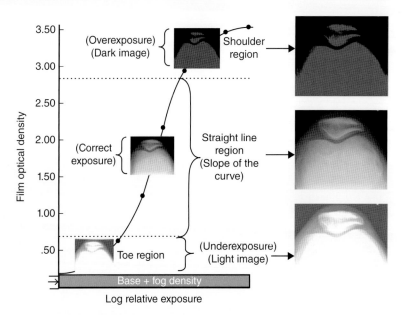

Figure 2.2 A plot of the OD as a function of the log of the relative radiation exposure is described by the well-known characteristic curve (Hurter–Driffield Curve), which provides information about the film response to the exposure. See text for further explanation.

here. The interested reader should refer to any standard radiography physics text for a further description of the other terms. While *film speed* refers to the sensitivity of the film to radiation and it is inversely proportional to the exposure, *film latitude* describes the range of exposures that would produce useful densities (contrast).

8. High-speed films (fast films) require less exposure than films with low speeds (slow films). On the other hand, while wide-exposure latitude films respond to a wide range of exposures, films with narrow exposure latitude can respond only to a small range of exposures. In the latter situation, the technologist has to be very precise in the selection of the exposure technique factors for examination.

A *significant limitation of FSR* that has been overcome by *digital radiography* (DR) relates to the narrow exposure latitude which means that exposure technique selection in FSR must be accurate to achieve an image with acceptable density and contrast. This poses a challenge as stated in point 8. For technologists, DR detectors "have wide exposure latitude, a variable speed class of operation, and image postprocessing capabilities that provide consistent image appearance even with underexposed or overexposed radiographs" [1]. This is illustrated in Figure 2.3. It is clear that DR images taken with low and high exposures appear visually the same on the viewing monitor (due to the image processing of DR systems). Note, however, while low exposures produce images with more noise (grainy image), high exposures produce images with less noise but at the expense of increased dose to the patient. The result is that technologists face a difficult task of recognizing underexposed and overexposed images. If overexposed images cannot be determined, the patient receives an unnecessary dose. Overexposures 5–10 times a normal exposure will appear acceptable to the technologist. Subsequently, this will lead to what has been popularly referred to as exposure creep or dose creep [1].

In FSR, the radiation exposure used for an examination is determined by the *exposure technique factors* selected on the radiographic control console by the technologist. These include

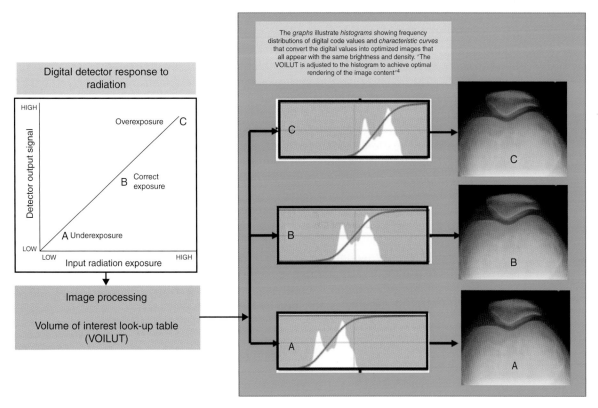

Figure 2.3 DR detectors have wide-exposure latitude and image postprocessing provides consistent image appearance even with underexposed or overexposed radiographs. See text for further explanation.

the kilovoltage (kV), the milliamperage (mA), and the time of exposure in seconds (s). Consoles may allow the selection of mAs (mA×s). While the kV determines the x-ray beam quality (beam penetration), the mA determines the quantity of photons falling on the patient per unit time. The length of time of the exposure is influenced by the exposure time. Today, automatic exposure control (AEC) is often used to ensure that correct exposure factors are used for examinations, and to reduce errors made by manual technique selection. The basic principle of an AEC timer is such when a preset quantity of radiation reaching the film detector (acceptable image density) is measured, the exposure is automatically terminated. The result is almost always perfect exposures.

Another essential concept in FSR is *image quality*. The quality of a film-based image can be described by several technical factors including resolution, contrast, noise, distortion, and artifacts. Only the first three will be reviewed in this chapter. Resolution includes two types, namely, spatial resolution and contrast resolution.

1. *Spatial resolution* refers to the detail or sharpness of the image, and is measured in line pairs/mm (lp/mm). The higher the number of lp/mm, the greater the sharpness of the image. FSR has the highest spatial resolution ranging from 5 to 15 lp/mm compared to all other imaging modalities [2]. As noted by Bushong [3], "Detail is affected by several factors such as the focal spot size, motion of the patient, and the image receptor design characteristics.

Detail is optimum when small focal spots are used, when the patient does not move during the exposure, and when detail cassettes are used."

2. *Contrast resolution* on the other hand describes the differences in tissue contrast that the film can show. As a radiation detector, film-screen cannot show differences in tissue contrast less than 10%. This means that film-based imaging is limited in its contrast resolution. For example, while the contrast resolution (mm at 0.5% difference) for FSR is 10, it is 20 for nuclear medicine, 10 for ultrasound, 4 for computed tomography (CT), and 1 for magnetic resonance imaging [2]. "The contrast of a radiographic film image, including the object, energy of the beam, scattered radiation, grids, and the film. The main controlling factor for image contrast, however, is kV. Optimum contrast is produced when low kV techniques are used. A grid improves radiographic contrast by absorbing scattered radiation before it gets to the film" [3].

3. *Noise* is seen on an image as having a grainy appearance. This occurs if few photons (quantity) are used to create the image. Noise can be reduced if more photons are used by using higher mAs settings; however, this will result in more dose to the patient. Less noise is produced when higher kV techniques are used for the same mA settings. The goal of the technologist is to use the lowest possible radiation dose and not compromise image quality. This is an important consideration in observing and working within the as low as reasonably achievable (ALARA) philosophy established by the ICRP.

DIGITAL RADIOGRAPHY MODALITIES: MAJOR SYSTEM COMPONENTS

Digital radiographic imaging systems generally referred to as DR has replaced the workhorse of diagnostic radiography, FSR. DR is defined by the American Association of Physicists in Medicine (AAPM) [4] as "radiographic imaging technology producing digital projection images such as those using photostimulable storage phosphor (computed radiography or CR), amorphous selenium, amorphous silicon, charge-coupled device (CCD), and metal oxide semiconductor-field effect transistor (MOSFET) technology." DR includes computed radiography (CR) and flat-panel digital radiography (FPDR); digital fluoroscopy (DF); digital mammography (DM); digital radiographic tomosynthesis (DRT) and digital breast tomosynthesis (DBT); and CT. These modalities are described in detail by Seeram [5].

The overall major system components of any DR modality are illustrated in Figure 2.4, and includes an x-ray generator, an x-ray tube, a digital detector, a computer, an image display monitor, and finally a digital communications system.

1. The x-ray generator provides the electrical power to the x-ray tube to provide the appropriate radiation exposure for the examination under investigation.
2. The patient is exposed and a latent image is created on the digital detector.
3. The latent image is processed by the computer and subsequently displayed on a monitor for viewing and interpretation.
4. The image can be stored and communicated to remote sites for viewing.

Each of the DR modalities listed above will be reviewed below with respect to major imaging system components only. The details of each of these modalities work will be described in later chapters.

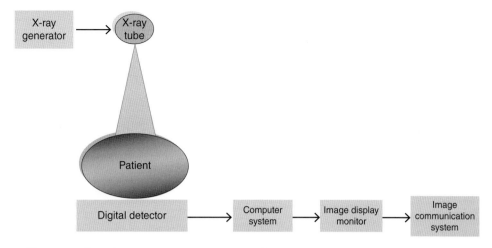

Figure 2.4   The overall major system components of any DR modality includes an x-ray generator, an x-ray tube, a digital detector, a computer, an image display monitor, and finally a digital communications system.

Computed radiography

The major components of a CR system are shown in Figure 2.5. These components include the imaging plate (IP), the IP processor, IP erasure, and image display monitor. After the IP is exposed as shown, a latent image is created on the IP. Subsequently, the IP is placed in the processor where it is scanned by a laser beam to render the latent image visible which is then displayed for viewing and interpretation. The IP is exposed to a bright light to erase any residual image, so that it can be used again.

Flat-panel digital radiography

The major system components of a FPDR system are shown in Figure 2.6 and include an x-ray generator, an x-ray tube, a flat-panel digital detector, a computer, an image display monitor, and finally a digital communications system.

The flat-panel digital detectors for FPDR fall into two categories, namely, the indirect conversion digital detector and the direct conversion digital detector. A significant difference between CR and FPDR systems is that the latter does not include a separate physical image reader but rather a digital processor is included in the design of the flat-panel detector, so that the latent image formed on the detector is subsequently rendered visible by the built-in digital processor. The image is then displayed on a monitor for viewing and interpretation.

Digital fluoroscopy

Fluoroscopy produces dynamic images acquired in *real-time* to allow for the study of motion of organ systems and hollow internal structures such as the gastrointestinal tract, as well as blood

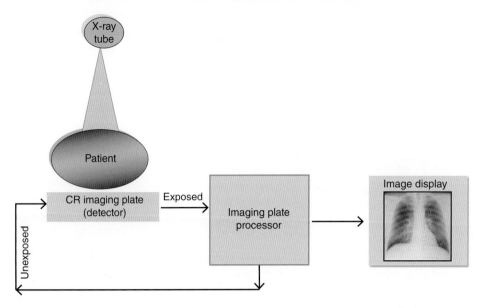

Figure 2.5   The major components of a CR system include the imaging plate (IP), the IP processor, IP erasure, and image display monitor.

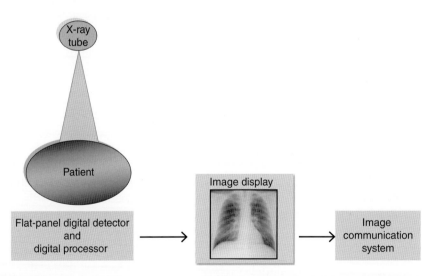

Figure 2.6   The major system components of a FPDR system include an x-ray generator, an x-ray tube, a flat-panel digital detector, a computer, an image display monitor, and finally a digital communications system.

circulatory system. The major system components of a DF system (Figure 2.7) consist of a flat-panel digital detector to allow for the creation of real-time dynamic images processed by a computer and subsequently displayed as a square image on the viewing monitor, compared to a circular image typical of the older image intensifier-based DF systems. This display method eliminates what is known as pin cushion distortion effects characteristic of the older digital fluoroscopic systems.

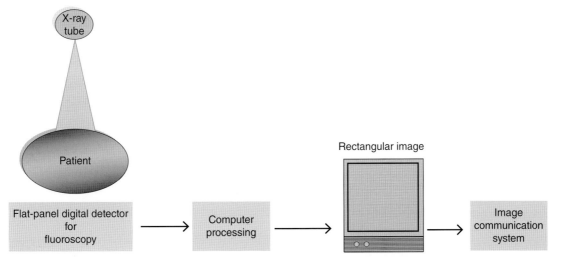

Figure 2.7 The major system components of a DF system consist of a flat-panel digital detector to allow for the creation of real-time dynamic images processed by a computer and subsequently display the image as a square image on the viewing monitor, compared to a circular image typical of the older image intensifier-based digital fluoroscopy systems. This display method eliminates what is known as pin cushion distortion effects characteristic of the older digital fluoroscopic systems.

Digital mammography

Major components of a DM system currently utilize CR detectors and flat-panel digital detectors including direct and indirect conversion detectors to image the breast. Image acquisition and processing is similar to that described above for FPDR. Additionally, associated applications of DM include DBT and DRT. While DBT is designed to examine only the breast, DRT images other body regions, such as the chest abdomen, extremities, for example. The basic concept of DBT and DRT is related to the principle underlying conventional tomography, in which the x-ray tube moves through various angles (limited arc) while the detector is stationary, capturing several images during the sweep, as illustrated in Figure 2.8. These images are subsequently subjected to image reconstruction algorithms and digital image processing to enhance the visualization of image features.

Computed tomography

CT is a *sectional imaging technique* that produces direct cross-sectional digital images referred to as transverse axial images. These images have been defined as planar sections that are perpendicular to the long axis of the patient. In CT, the patient is scanned as the x-ray tube coupled to special electronic detectors rotate around the patient to collect and measure attenuation readings as shown in Figure 2.9. Furthermore, the raw data from the detectors are sent to a computer which uses an image reconstruction algorithm to build up images of the anatomy scanned. These images are subsequently displayed for viewing and interpretation, after which they are sent to an image communication system for storage, archiving, and communication to various remote locations, if needed.

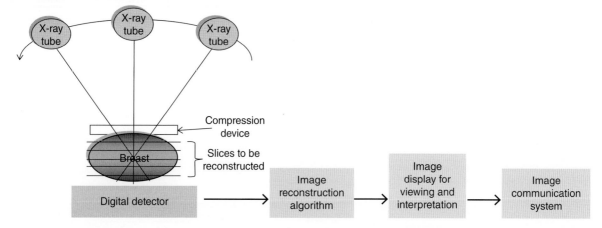

Figure 2.8　The basic concept for DBT and DRT is related to the principle underlying conventional tomography, in which the x-ray tube moves through various angles (limited arc) while the detector is stationary, capturing several images during the sweep. See text for further explanation.

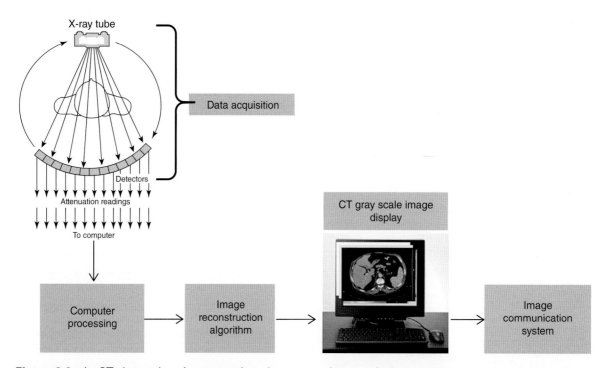

Figure 2.9　In CT, the patient is scanned as the x-ray tube coupled to special electronic detectors rotate around the patient to collect and measure attenuation readings as illustrated.

IMAGE COMMUNICATION SYSTEMS

Image communication systems include picture archiving and communication systems (PACS) and information systems, including hospital information systems (HIS) and radiology information systems (RIS); Cloud PACS, a technology derived from cloud computing; Vendor Neutral Archives (VNAs); and Enterprise Imaging.

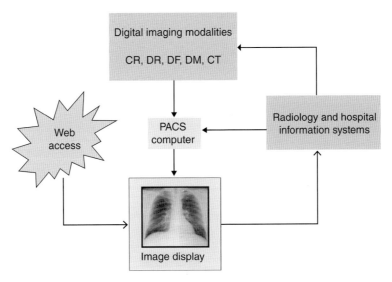

Figure 2.10   The major system components of a PACS make use of digital technologies for storage, display, and communication of digital images acquired by all digital modalities. Furthermore, a computer system performs tasks of image storage, archiving, and image processing.

Picture archiving and communication system

The PACS is a significant component in a DR environment. A PACS makes use of digital technologies for storage, display, and communication of digital images acquired by all digital modalities. As illustrated in Figure 2.10, the system consists of a number of components such as a computer system that performs tasks of image storage, archiving, and image processing. Coupled to a large-scale PACS are the *information systems*: the RIS and the HIS. Furthermore, the PACS can be accessed via the Internet as well.

Image communication systems continue to evolve into systems intended to improve the performance of PACS. These technologies include *Cloud PACS*, a technology derived from *cloud computing*; *VNAs*; and *Enterprise Imaging*. These systems are described in detail by Seeram [5].

References

1. Seibert, J.A. and Morin, R.L. (2011). The standardized exposure index for digital radiography: an opportunity for optimization of radiation dose to the pediatric population. *Pediatr. Radiol.* 41: 573–581.
2. Seeram, E., Davidson, R., Bushong, S., and Swan, H. (2016). Optimizing the exposure indicator as a dose management strategy in computed radiography. *Radiol. Technol.* 87 (4): 380–391.
3. Bushong, S. (2020). *Radiologic Science for Technologists*, 12e. St. Louis, MO: Elsevier (in Press).
4. American Association of Physicists in Medicine (AAPM) (2009). An Exposure Indicator for Digital Radiography. College Park, MD: AAPM. *Report No. 116*.
5. Seeram, E. (2019). *Digital Radiography: Physical Principles and Quality Control*, 2e. Singapore: Springer Nature Singapore Pte Ltd.

SECTION 2

Basic Radiographic Sciences and Technology

3

Basic physics of diagnostic radiography

In Chapter 2, the essential principles of film-screen radiography (FSR) were reviewed as a basis of providing a rationale for the introduction of digital radiography (DR) modalities. Furthermore, the general system components of computed radiography (CR) and flat-panel digital radiography (FPDR); digital fluoroscopy (DF); digital mammography (DM); digital radiographic tomosynthesis

A Comprehensive Guide to Radiographic Sciences and Technology, First Edition. Euclid Seeram.
© 2021 John Wiley & Sons Ltd. Published 2021 by John Wiley & Sons Ltd.

(DRT) and digital breast tomosynthesis (DBT); and computed tomography (CT) were identified. The goal of Chapter 2 was to identify the major components and more importantly to lay the foundations needed for a good understanding of how each component works to create images and protect not only patients but technologists as well.

The purpose of this chapter is to briefly identify and explain the relevant physics concepts that are common to all diagnostic imaging modalities, particularly in creating images and managing the radiation dose to patients. The physics topics that will be reviewed in this chapter include the structure of the atom, the nature of radiation, x-ray generation and production, x-ray emission, attenuation of radiation, and the interaction of x-ray with matter. Other related physical factors are direct and indirect action of radiation, radiolysis of water, linear energy transfer and relative biological effectiveness. The latter topics are essential to a further grasp of radiobiology; that is, the effects of radiation on biological systems.

STRUCTURE OF THE ATOM

The production of x-rays to image the patient in diagnostic radiography requires an understanding of the structure of matter, which is made up of atoms, the building blocks of the universe. Furthermore, when a beam of x-rays passes through the body, x-ray photons in the beam interact with first, the atoms that make up the various tissues of the patient and second, the atoms that make up the structure of the detector, which creates a latent image. These are only two examples why it is important for technologists to understand the nature of *atomic structure*.

Nucleus

A simple model of the atom illustrated in Figure 3.1 shows a central dense *nucleus* which is positively charged and which consists of two particles: *protons* (positively charged) and *neutrons* (no charge) surrounded by *electrons* (negatively charged). The number of protons in the nucleus is called the *atomic number* (Z), and the total number of protons and neutrons (nucleons) is called the *mass number* (A), not to be confused with the *atomic mass*, the actual mass of the atom.

Electrons, quantum levels, binding energy, electron volts

Depending on the atom, electrons orbit the nucleus at fixed distances in different orbital levels referred to as *quantum levels* or orbits, or *shells* (so-called because the orbits are three-dimensional) represented by the letters K, L, M, N, O. . . with the K shell being the innermost shell (closest to the nucleus). These shells are also assigned corresponding quantum numbers (1, 2, 3, 4, 5. . .) with the K shell being assigned a quantum number of 1. The number of electrons contained in each shell is given by the expression $2(n)^2$, where n is the quantum number of the shell. For example, the K shell can only contain two electrons [$2 \times (1)^2$] while the M shell can have only 18 electrons, and so on. Electrons are held in their respective orbits by an electromagnetic force (due to the electrostatic pull of the positively charged nucleus) known as the *binding energy*. Electrons can only be removed from their orbits if the energy of an incoming particle or x-ray photon is greater than the binding energy. Furthermore, outermost shell electrons known as the valence electrons (responsible for the chemical properties of the atom) are most easily removed from the atom. The binding energy can be expressed as *electron volts* (eV).

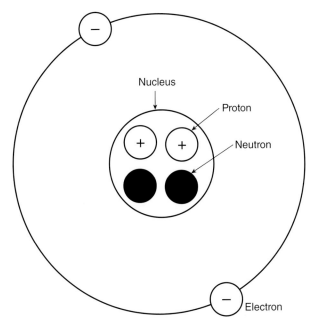

Figure 3.1 Bohr's planetary model of the atom shows a dense nucleus surrounded by orbiting electrons.

For example, while the inner shell electron binding energy is thousands of electron volts (keV), that of the outer shell is equal to about several eVs. Additionally, as the number of protons in the nucleus increases, the binding energy increases as well. This means that the binding energy for a hydrogen (Z = 1) K shell electron is less than that of a tungsten (Z = 74) K shell electron.

Electrons can be transferred to other shells within the atom or they can be completely removed from the atom. The removal of an electron from its orbit creates a vacancy, or hole, in that orbit. This prompts a cascading effect in which the hole is filled immediately by an electron from an outer orbit, and so on down through successively affected orbits. In other words, if a K-shell electron is ejected, an electron from the L-shell may fill the vacancy in the K-shell, the L-shell vacancy may be filled with an electron from the M-shell, and so on. The energy released by these electron transitions is expressed in one of two ways: as electromagnetic or particulate radiation. The major characteristics of each of these two types of radiation will be reviewed later in this chapter.

ENERGY DISSIPATION IN MATTER

Excitation

In *excitation*, a fraction of the energy of the radiation is transferred to the electrons of the absorbing material. Electrons respond by jumping to another orbital level farther away from the nucleus. They are not ejected from the atom. This is illustrated in Figure 3.2, where the K-shell electron is raised to the L-shell as the positive charge passes the atom. As the positive charge moves away from the atom, the electron falls back into its original orbit.

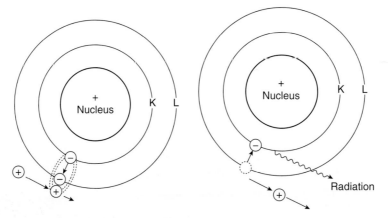

Figure 3.2 During excitation of the atom, electrons are not ejected, but rather, they are moved into orbital levels that are farther away from the central nucleus.

Ionization

In contrast to excitation, *ionization* occurs when the radiation has enough energy to eject the electron completely from the atom. In other words, the amount of energy is greater than the binding energy of the electron. In this case, the radiation is referred to as *ionizing radiation*. Every ionization event results in an energy dissipation of ~33 eV, the amount of energy needed to break chemical bonds.

Ionization results in *ion pairs*, which are made up of the ejected electron (negative ion) and the portion of the atom that remains (positive ion) after loss of the electron.

Depending on its energy, the ejected electron can cause further ionization along the length of the path it travels in the absorbing material. This process, referred to as *secondary ionization*, gives rise to secondary electrons or "delta rays."

TYPES OF RADIATION

Earlier reference was made to both *electromagnetic* and *particulate radiations*, the types of radiation that appear as a result of the energy released by electron transitions. In this section, the essential characteristics will be briefly reviewed. The student who is interested in a more thorough treatment of these topics should refer to a radiologic physics textbook, such as one by Bushberg et al. [1].

Radiation is the propagation of energy through space or matter, in the form of waves or particles. In general, there are two types of radiation: *natural background radiation* and *human-made radiation* (formerly referred to as man-made). An example of the former type is cosmic radiation, which consists of high-speed particles that originate in space. Cosmic radiation bombards the Earth, and nothing can be done to stop it. The Earth itself consists of various sources of natural radiation, such as rocks, water, granite, natural gas, the air, and phosphates. Even our bodies emit some form of radiation. Human-made radiation arises from nuclear reactors, nuclear fallout, and artificially produced materials. In diagnostic x-ray imaging, the source of x-rays is the x-ray tube. Radiation, whether it be natural or human-made, falls into two classes: electromagnetic radiation and particulate radiation.

Electromagnetic radiation

Electromagnetic radiation consists of both an electric and a magnetic field propagating through space at right angles to each other. These fields are capable of energy transfer from point to point and have physical properties that are similar to those of visible light. There are several forms of electromagnetic radiation and these include cosmic rays (high energy, short wavelength), gamma rays, x-rays, ultraviolet radiation, visible light, infrared (heat) radiation, microwaves, and radio-waves (low energy, long wavelength). These radiations are arranged systematically to show the range of their frequencies, wavelengths, and energies in an arrangement known as the *electromagnetic spectrum* (EMS).

The different types of electromagnetic radiation can be described in terms of their energy and wavelength. The energy of the radiation is inversely proportional to the wavelength. This means that the higher the energy, the shorter the wavelength, and the more penetrating its radiation. For example, x-rays and gamma rays are more penetrating than ultraviolet light, which can penetrate the human skin to only about 1 mm.

X-rays and gamma rays are both classified as *ionizing radiation*. That is to say, each type of radiation interacts with matter so as to eject electrons completely from the atom, thus leaving behind *ion pairs*. Ultraviolet radiation, visible light, infrared radiation, microwaves, and radio-waves belong to the class of *nonionizing radiation*, which means that they do not have enough energy to eject electrons from the atom.

Wave–particle duality

Electromagnetic radiation can be thought of as having a *wave–particle duality*, meaning that the radiation can behave physically either as a wave as a particle. While a *wave* is a disturbance that carries energy from point to point, a *particle* is a discrete "packet" of energy referred to as a *quantum* called a *photon*. Photons are responsible for ejecting electrons from atoms, thus resulting in ionization.

A wave is characterized by its velocity, wavelength, and frequency. The frequency (f) refers to the number of vibrations per second and its unit of measurement is cycles per second (cps). The unit can also be given in hertz (Hz), where 1 Hz = 1 cps. The wavelength (λ) is the distance taken up by 1 cycle of a wave. The unit of wavelength is meter (m).

The fundamental wave equation relates λ and f of a wave to its speed or velocity (c) as:

$$c = \lambda f. \tag{3.1}$$

X-rays can behave as waves or as particles. It was Max Planck who suggested that these photons had an energy (E) related to the frequency (υ) in the following algebraic expression:

$$E = h\upsilon, \tag{3.2}$$

where h is a constant known as Planck's constant (h = 6.626×10^{-34} Js). The relationship between E and λ (in nanometers nm), on the other hand, is given by the algebraic expression:

$$E(keV) = 1.24 / \lambda. \tag{3.3}$$

The unit of energy, E, is the electron volt (eV) which is the energy acquired by one electron as it travels under a potential difference of 1 V in a vacuum. In diagnostic imaging, E is expressed in kiloelectron volts (keV, where 1 keV = 1000 V). In Eq. (3.3), the unit of wavelength (λ) is the angstrom (Å) which is equal to 10^{-8} cm.

Particulate radiation

Particulate radiation refers to particles that are ejected from atoms at very high speeds, and have, in most cases, extremely high energies. Particulate radiation may include one or more components of the atom, such as the electron, proton, or a neutron. Examples of particulate radiation are alpha particles (helium nuclei), beta particles [electrons, protons (positively charged particles)], energetic neutrons (atomic particles with no charge), and cosmic radiation.

The penetrating power of these particles varies. For example, alpha particles are less penetrating than beta particles, which are in turn less penetrating than x-rays or gamma rays. A thin sheet of paper will shield against alpha particles, whereas beta particles will penetrate the paper, but may be shielded by a block of wood.

X-RAY GENERATION

There are three major parts to an x-ray imaging system, and each consists of an electrical circuit; the circuit that comprise the *x-ray operator control console*, the *high-voltage generator circuit*, and the *x-ray tube circuit*. While the high-voltage circuit and x-ray tube circuits are located in what is referred to the high-voltage section of the complete circuit, the operator console circuit is located in the low-voltage section of the complete circuit. The purpose of the operator control console is to provide an interface between the electronics of the imaging system and the patient. This means that this circuit allows the technologist to select the essential technical factors (for example, the kV, mAs, and the specific exposure timing mechanism, such as automatic exposure control) needed to produce the appropriate x-rays from the x-ray tube for the examination under study.

X-rays are produced when high-speed electrons strike a target. To obtain the necessary high speeds, the *x-ray generator* provides the high voltage (thousands of volts = kV) to the x-ray tube in order to obtain the intensity of x-rays needed for the examination under investigation. Furthermore, the generator consists of several electrical components to change the electrical power from the utility company into a form suitable for x-ray production and control. These two components are transformers and rectifiers.

Transformers can be step-up or step-down devices. While the former increases the low voltage from the utility company (120 or 220 V for example) to high voltage (say from 25 to 150 kV), which is a requirement for producing x-rays, the latter decreases the current and the voltage from the utility company to levels suitable for energizing the x-ray tube. *Rectifiers* are electrical devices which are part of the generator circuit that change the alternating current (AC) from the utility company into a direct current (DC) through a process known as rectification. *Rectification* allows the electrons in the x-ray tube to flow only in one direction, that is, from cathode to anode, another important requirement for x-ray production. Further essential characteristics of the x-ray tube and the circuits comprising the x-ray imaging system (low voltage and high voltage sections) will be reviewed in Chapter 4.

X-RAY PRODUCTION

X-rays were discovered by Professor WC Roentgen in 1895, while he was researching the nature of cathode rays (electrons). During his experiments, he noticed the fluorescence of a barium–platinocyanide screen located near the cathode ray tube with which he was working.

He attributed this fluorescence to something (that was invisible) coming from the tube. He called this something, *x-rays*. Further experiments led him to see the bones of his hands when he placed them between the tube and the screen. Not only were these rays invisible, they were penetrating as well.

Properties of x-rays

Roentgen's early experiments led him to several conclusions about the properties of x-rays, several of which include the following:

1. X-rays can affect photographic plates.
2. X-rays are not affected by electrical or magnetic fields.
3. X-rays can cause certain materials to fluoresce.
4. X-rays can cause ionization.
5. X-rays can be absorbed by high atomic number elements such as lead.
6. X-rays can penetrate most substances, including soft tissues and bone.

These properties make x-rays particularly suitable for use in diagnostic radiology.

Origin of x-rays

As stated earlier, x-rays are produced when high-speed electrons strike a target. In an x-ray tube, these electrons come from the filament of the cathode, and are accelerated across the vacuum in the tube, to strike the nuclei of the target atoms of the anode. There are two important considerations to note in this regard:

1. When the interaction is between high-speed electrons and the inner shell electrons of the anode target atoms, *characteristic x-rays* are produced.
2. When the interaction is between high-speed electrons and the charged nuclei of the anode target atoms, *Bremsstrahlung* x-rays are produced.

Characteristic radiation

The production of characteristic x-rays is illustrated in Figure 3.3. When high-speed electrons interact with inner shell electrons of the anode target atoms to cause ionization, characteristic radiation results. As the electrons move from any of the outer shells to replace electrons ejected from the inner shell, x-ray photons are produced. In Figure 3.3, the electron from the L-shell fills the K-shell vacancy, resulting in the production of x-rays. Characteristic x-rays are only useful in diagnostic radiology if they have enough energy to penetrate body tissues and fall upon the image receptor (detector).

X-rays emitted as a result of the K-shell being filled are called K-characteristic x-rays. Similarly, L-characteristic x-rays, M-characteristic x-rays, and so on, can be produced. These emissions are called characteristic because the x-rays produced are characteristic of target elements, and differ as a function of their binding energy. For example, the energy of K-characteristic x-rays of a tungsten target will be different from the energy of K-characteristic x-rays of a lead target.

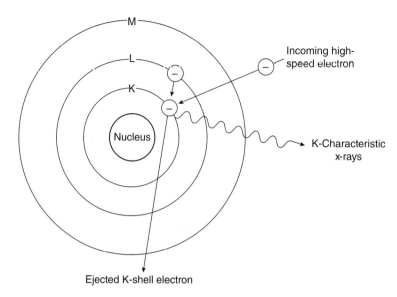

Figure 3.3   The production of characteristic radiation.

Bremsstrahlung radiation

Bremsstrahlung is the German word for "braking" or "slowing down." Brems (for short) radiation is produced when a high-speed electron is decelerated in an interaction with the charged nuclei of target atoms (and not the electrons). As an electron approaches the nucleus, it slows down, loses its initial kinetic energy (KE) and changes its direction of travel, with less KE. The difference in KE reappears in the form of Bremsstrahlung radiation as shown in Figure 3.4. Brems radiation can have a wide range of energies, because the incoming high-speed electrons can lose varying amounts of KE as they pass by the nucleus. Those that are closer to the nucleus will cause an emission of relatively *high-energy x-rays*, while those that are farther away from the nucleus will emit relatively *low-energy x-rays*. *Medium-energy x-rays* fall in between the two. For example, a high-speed electron with a KE of 70 keV can result in Brems radiation having energies ranging from 0 to 70 keV. Recall that characteristic x-rays can be produced only at specific energies equal to the difference in the binding energies of the electrons in the inner and outer shells.

X-RAY EMISSION

The emission of characteristic and Brems radiation is illustrated in Figure 3.5. This is referred to as the *x-ray emission spectrum*, which is a plot of the number of x-ray photons per unit energy (intensity) as a function of x-ray energy. An understanding of the x-ray emission spectrum will provide the technologist with a further insight into how various technical factors (such as, for example, kV, mA, filtration, voltage waveform, and target material of the x-ray tube) affect the radiation dose to the patient. These will be reviewed subsequently.

Two emission spectra are shown in Figure 3.5: the characteristic or *discrete emission spectrum*, and the Brems or *continuous emission spectrum*. Whereas the discrete spectrum shows that characteristic x-rays are emitted only at specific photon energies, the continuous spectrum shows that the energies of Brems radiation range from 0 to some maximum value. The maximum energy of emitted x-rays is numerically equal to the kVp used for the examination. This is why it is called kV**p(eak)** [2].

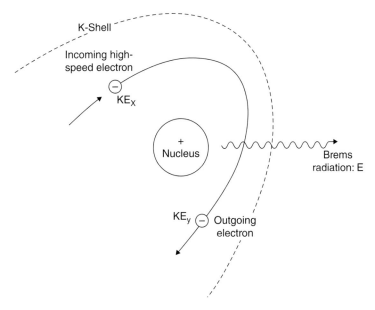

Figure 3.4   Bremsstrahlung radiation is produced when a high-speed electron is decelerated in an interaction with the charged nuclei of target atoms.

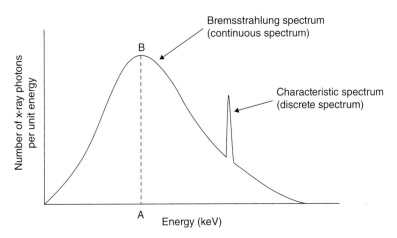

Figure 3.5   The general form and shape of both the discrete and continuous x-ray spectra. The line AB represents the amplitude of the continuous spectrum. See text for further explanation.

X-RAY BEAM QUANTITY AND QUALITY

The number of x-ray photons in the beam per unit energy, that is, the area under the curve of the emission spectrum, is called the x-ray beam *quantity*. The quantity of x-rays increased when the current (amperes) to the filament of the x-ray tube is increased; this of course translates into an increase in filament temperature. As the filament temperature increases, more electrons are produced. More electrons simply mean more x-rays, and therefore, an increase in quantity. There are other factors affecting x-ray quantity, and these include the x-ray tube current (mA, which is not the filament current), the tube voltage (kV), beam filtration, the distance from the target of the tube to the image receptor, and the atomic number of the target material. These factors affect the size and relative position of the x-ray emission spectrum.

The *quality* of the x-ray beam refers to the energy of the beam. In this case, the energy of the beam is sometimes discussed as "hardness" or "penetrating power." Beam quality is controlled by the voltage (kV) applied between the anode and cathode of the x-ray tube. Increasing the kV across the tune increases the beam energy, since the electrons from the filament are accelerated across the tube with more KE. Other factors that affect the quality of the x-ray beam include the target material, filtration, and the voltage waveforms. These factors affecting quantity and quality will be described briefly in the following section.

Factors affecting x-ray beam quantity and quality

This section is devoted to examining how these factors (as stated above) affect the size and relative position of both the continuous and discrete x-ray spectra. The technologist has direct control of two of these factors, the kV and the mA or mAs.

kV
The higher the kV, the greater the beam quality. Higher kV will also affect the beam intensity (I) through the following algebraic expression:

$$I \alpha \left(kV\right)^2.$$ (3.4)

This implies that as the kV is doubled, the intensity will increase by a factor of four. Intensity problems can be solved using the following algebraic expression:

$$I_1 / I_2 = \left(kV_1 / kV_2\right)^2,$$ (3.5)

where I_1 and I_2 are intensities at kV_1 and kV_2, respectively.

An increase in kV will alter the spectrum by increasing the amplitude, or height of the wave, of the continuous spectrum (the area under the curve is increased) as illustrated in Figure 3.6. Note that the amplitude is increased and the position of the spectrum is shifted toward higher energies. The discrete spectrum remains the same because it is not influenced by the kV.

mA
The tube current (mA) determines the quantity of photons because it affects the number of electrons flowing from the filament to the target of the x-ray tube. The greater the mA, the greater the number of electrons and the greater the quantity of x-rays. The quantity of x-rays is directly proportional to the mA, that is:

$$I \alpha \, mA.$$ (3.6)

If the mA is doubled, the quantity of x-rays doubles as shown in Figure 3.7. Note that, while the amplitude changes proportionately, the position of the continuous spectrum does not shift toward higher energies. The discrete spectrum is not influenced by the mA. The same holds true for mAs (milliamperage-seconds).

Target material
The atomic number (Z) of the target material of the tube affects both the quantity and quality of the x-ray beam, such that the higher the Z of the target material, the more efficient is the

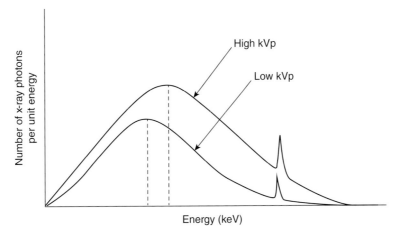

Figure 3.6 The effect of kV on the intensity and quality of x-rays. Note that the discrete spectrum remains at the same position on the energy axis, while the amplitude of the continuous spectrum shifts to the higher energy region. The continuous spectrum increases in amplitude for high kV techniques.

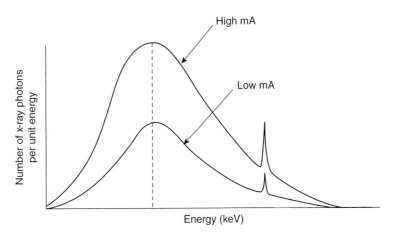

Figure 3.7 The effects of mA on x-ray spectra. The area under the curve increases proportionally as the mA increases. There is no shift of the amplitude on the photon energy axis, indicating that mA does not affect the beam energy.

production of Brems radiation. This means that the amplitude of the continuous spectrum is increased (increased in quantity) as the Z of the target material increases (Figure 3.8). Note now, that there is a change in the position of the discrete spectrum. The Z of the target material influences the quality of the characteristic radiation.

X-ray beam filtration

The x-ray beam from the x-ray tube is a heterogeneous radiation beam comprised of low-energy and high-energy photons. A filter placed in the x-ray beam is intended to preferentially absorb the low-energy photons which are less likely to reach the image receptor. These photons only increase the dose to the patient. With the removal of low-energy photons, the beam becomes harder or more penetrating, that is, the mean energy of the beam increases. Filtration therefore is intended to protect the patient.

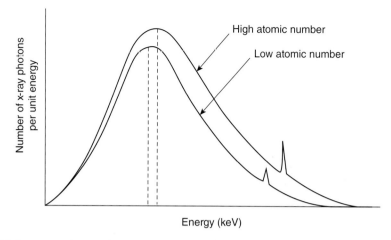

Figure 3.8   For higher atomic number target materials, there is an increase in quantity as well as quality of the x-ray beam compared with target materials of lower atomic number. Note there is a change in the position of the discrete spectrum.

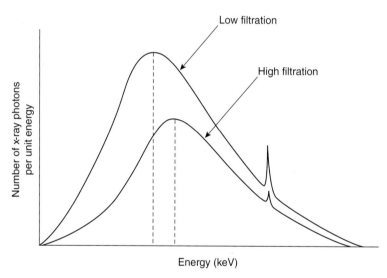

Figure 3.9   The effect of filtration on the x-ray spectra. For high filtration, there is a reduction in the intensity of the beam and an increase in the beam energy (amplitude of the continuous spectrum shifts to the right on the energy axis). The position of the discrete spectrum remains the same.

An increase in filtration will change the shape and position of the continuous spectrum, but leaves the discrete spectrum unaffected. Figure 3.9 shows that for a constant kV and mA, an increase in filtration will result in a decrease in x-ray intensity (area under the curve) and an increase in the effective energy of the x-ray beam.

Voltage waveform

The voltage waveform for the generation of x-rays depends on the type of generator. The type of generator affects the continuous spectrum, but not the discrete spectrum, as illustrated in Figure 3.10. This will be described further in Chapter 4.

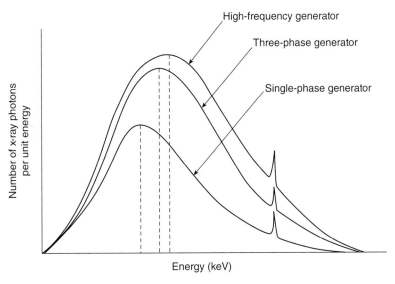

Figure 3.10 The effect of rectification on the x-ray spectra. For three-phase and high-frequency generators, both the intensity and the effective energy on the beam increase.

A general relationship

The general relationship between intensity (I) and kV, mA, and atomic number is expressed in the following algebraic expression:

$$I \, \alpha \, kV^2 \times mA \times Z. \tag{3.7}$$

This relationship is one of direct proportionality which means that:

1. Intensity increases proportionately as the mA increases.
2. Intensity increases proportionately as the square of the kV.
3. Intensity increases proportionately as the Z of the target material increases.

If the distance from the x-ray tube to the image receptor is introduced as another factor, then the expression (Eq. 3.7) becomes:

$$I \, \alpha \, kV^2 \times mA \times Z \, / \, d^2. \tag{3.8}$$

The intensity is inversely proportional to the square of the distance. High kV and low mA exposure techniques result in a decreased dose to the patient.

INTERACTION OF RADIATION WITH MATTER

When radiation interacts with matter, some of the photons of the beam will be absorbed (*absorption*), some will be scattered (*scattering*), and some will penetrate the material (*penetration*). These processes depend on the energy of the photons as well as on the composition of the absorbing material, and contribute to the reduction of the number of photons (intensity) in the beam. This reduction is referred to as attenuation. The intricacies of this phenomenon will be explored subsequently. It is important at this stage, however, to consider different mechanisms by which x-rays interact with matter. Because x-rays can have a range of energies (low, moderate, and high), there are five different mechanisms of interaction: (i) classical or Rayleigh scattering, (ii) Compton scattering, (iii) photoelectric absorption or photoelectric effect as it is sometimes referred to, (iv) pair production, and (v) photodisintegration. In this section, only the first three will be reviewed since they occur in diagnostic x-ray imaging. Since pair production and photodisintegration occur at very high energies beyond those used in diagnostic imaging, they will not be described in this book. The reader may refer to Bushong [2] and Bushberg et al. [1] for descriptions of these two processes.

Mechanisms of interaction in diagnostic x-ray imaging

When the absorbing material has many atoms in a small volume, then the chance of an interaction is greater than when there are few atoms encompassed within the same volume. The chance that an interaction will occur is referred to as its *probability*. The probability that a given interaction will occur depends upon a number of factors, including the atomic number (Z) of the absorbing material and the energy of the photons.

Classical scattering

When a low-energy photon (about 10 keV) interacts with an atom, it is absorbed by the entire atom. There is no ionization, but the atom becomes excited and very quickly releases a photon with energy equal to that of the incident photon. The released photon is scattered in a different direction as shown in Figure 3.11. For energies used in diagnostic radiography, less than 5% of x-ray interactions are due to *classical scattering*. This percentage contributes very little to image formation. Classical scattering is also referred to as elastic or Rayleigh scattering.

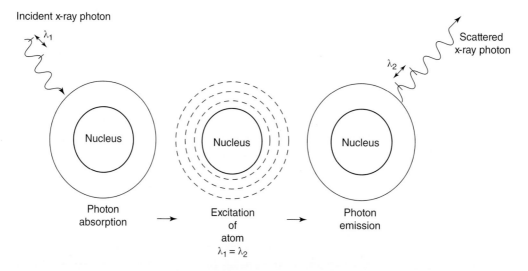

Figure 3.11 Classical scattering. A low-energy photon is absorbed by the atom resulting in excitation. This excitation quickly releases a photon with energy equal to that of the incident photon.

Compton scattering

Another photon–electron interaction that is of vital importance to the technologist is *Compton scattering* (also referred to as inelastic or nonclassical scattering) because it is the predominant interaction in x-ray imaging. In Compton scattering (Figure 3.12), an incident photon interacts with electrons in the outer shell of the atom. The incident photon has enough energy to eject the electron from its shell, resulting in ionization of the atom. The incident photon is scattered in a different direction, which is defined by the angle of deflection. The following points should be noted with respect to Compton scattering:

1. The energy of the scattered photon is less than the energy of the incident photon.
2. After the collision, the energy of the incident photon is distributed between the energy of the scattered photon and that of the ejected electron. For a 70 keV incident photon, the energy of the scattered photon is large when the scattering angle is small.

The probability that Compton scattering will occur depends on the energy of the incident photon, and the electron density (number of electrons per gram of absorber × density). As the energy of the incident photon and the density of the absorber increase, the probability of Compton scattering increases. The probability of Compton scattering does not depend on the atomic number of the absorber. It is important to note that during a diagnostic exposure, both Compton

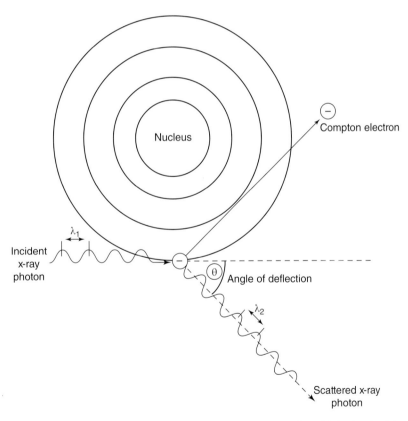

Figure 3.12 Compton scattering is a photon–electron interaction in which the incident photon interacts with electrons in the outer shell of the atom, resulting in a high-speed electron and scattered x-rays.

scattering and another interaction mechanism, photoelectric absorption, will occur. The one that predominates depends on the kV used for the examination. Generally, Compton scattering predominates at higher kV techniques (lower tissue contrast) and photoelectric absorption predominates at lower kV techniques (higher tissue contrast). For FSR, this would mean that lower kV techniques result in greater image contrast, while at higher kV techniques would result in lower image contrast.

Photoelectric absorption

Photoelectric absorption (photoelectric effect) is another x-ray interaction mechanism with matter. This is schematically shown in Figure 3.13. The incident photon interacts with inner shell electrons (K or L) and transfers all of its energy to these electrons. The electron absorbs this energy and is ejected from the atom (Figure 3.13). The ejected electron is referred to as a photoelectron. The vacancy now left in the inner shell is filled by an electron in the neighboring outer shell, resulting in characteristic x-ray emission. The energy of the photoelectron is equal to the energy of the incident photon minus the binding energy of the ejected electron.

Photoelectric absorption results in:

1. photoelectron
2. ionization of the atom (what remains after the electron is ejected is a positive ion)
3. characteristic x-rays

The probability of occurrence of photoelectric absorption depends on the atomic number of the absorber and the energy of the incident photon, and is greatest with high atomic number elements and low energy radiation. Thus, bone has an effective Z of 13.8 and will absorb more radiation than soft tissue, which has an effective Z of 7.4. Furthermore, because the probability of photoelectric absorption is inversely proportional to the energy of the incident photons. Increasing this energy by a factor of 2, photoelectric absorption decreases by a factor of 8. Photoelectric absorption is responsible for much of the high contrast in x-ray imaging, because it results in complete absorption of the photon, and therefore contributes significantly to the radiation dose to the patient.

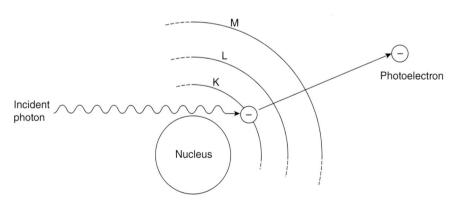

Figure 3.13 Photoelectric absorption occurs when an incident photon interacts with inner shell electrons of the atom. The electron ejected from the atom is referred to as a photoelectron. The vacancy left in the inner shell is filled by an electron in a neighboring outer shell resulting in the production of characteristic x-rays.

RADIATION ATTENUATION

Attenuation is the reduction of the intensity of radiation as it passes through matter. The interactions or mechanisms just described are examples of how radiation is attenuated, by both absorption and scattering.

Linear attenuation coefficient

When a beam of radiation passes through material, a fraction of the photons is removed from the beam per unit thickness of the material. This is referred to as the linear attenuation coefficient (μ) and its unit is the inverse centimeter (cm^{-1}). For a small thickness Δx, the number of photons removed is given by the algebraic expression:

$$n = \mu N \Delta x, \tag{3.9}$$

where n is the number of photons removed and N is the original number of photons entering the material. As the thickness of the material increases, Eq. (3.9) does not hold true. Bushberg et al. [1] states that "for a monoenergetic beam of photons incident upon either thick or thin slabs of material, an exponential relationship exists between the number of incident photons (N_0) and those that are transmitted (N) through a thickness x, without interaction:

$$N = N_0 e^{-\mu x}." \tag{3.10}$$

The factors affecting the linear attenuation coefficient include the following: (i) the energy of the beam, (ii) the atomic number and density of the absorbing material, and (iii) the electrons per gram of absorber. Increasing the energy of the beam (going from 90 to 120 kV) increases the number of transmitted photons and hence decreases attenuation. Increasing the density, Z, and electrons per gram of the absorber, leads to a decrease in the number of transmitted photons, thus leading to an increase in attenuation. For example, lead (Z = 82) will attenuate more radiation than gold (Z = 79).

In general, and with respect to radiation attenuation and dose in particular, the technologist should consider the following when imaging patients:

1. High kV exposure techniques decrease attenuation.
2. Low kV exposure techniques increase attenuation.
3. Bone attenuates more radiation than soft tissues because of its higher atomic number.
4. The probability of photoelectric absorption is seven times greater in bone than in soft tissues regardless of energy [2].
5. As the density (mass per unit volume) of the tissue increases, attenuation increases.
6. Contrast media (containing iodine or barium for example) will attenuate more radiation than soft tissues because of their higher Z and densities, particularly at low kV exposure techniques.

Mass attenuation coefficient

Another measure of radiation attenuation is the *mass attenuation coefficient* defined as the linear attenuation coefficient (μ) divided by the density (ρ) of the material, and "use of the mass attenuation coefficient allows attenuation to be described as a function of the mass of the material traversed rather than the physical distance" [3]. While the unit of the linear attenuation coefficient is cm^{-1}, the unit of the mass attenuation coefficient is cm^2/gram (g). As noted by Bushberg et al. [1] ". . .in radiology, we do not usually compare equal masses. Instead, we usually compare regions of an image that corresponds to irradiation of adjacent volumes of tissue. Therefore, density, the mass contained within a given volume plays an important role. Thus, one can radiographically visualize ice in a cup of water due to the density difference between the ice and the water."

The mass thickness (g/cm^2 or $\rho \times t$) can be used to specify the thickness of the absorber and this is used to calculate the attenuation using the value of the mass attenuation coefficient as follows: attenuation = $(\rho \times t) \times (\mu/\rho)$ [3].

Half value layer

A practical measure of the attenuation is the *half value layer* (HVL) which is defined as the thickness of material needed to reduce the intensity of the radiation beam by 50%. The HVL expresses the quality, or penetrating power, of the beam.

For a homogeneous beam of radiation, in which all the photons have the same energy, equal thicknesses of material will remove the same percentage of photons from the beam. The energy of the transmitted photons remains the same, but there is a decrease in the quantity of photons. This is not the same with a heterogeneous beam in which photons have different energies. The beam from the x-ray tube is a heterogeneous beam, and therefore it is important to consider what happens to such a beam as it passes through matter. For a heterogeneous beam, equal thicknesses of material remove different amounts of photons from the beam. The transmitted beam has a higher effective energy than the incident beam, because the low-energy photons have been absorbed or filtered by the material. This is known as *beam hardening*. Attenuation mechanisms for a homogeneous beam and a heterogeneous beam are illustrated in Figure 3.14.

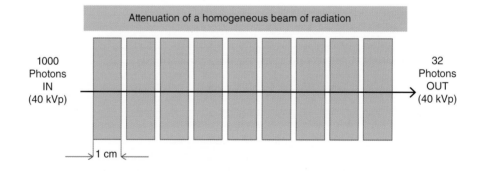

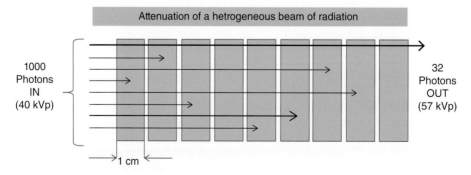

Figure 3.14 The difference between the attenuation of a homogeneous beam and a heterogeneous beam of radiation. See text for further explanation.

The radiation beam from the x-ray tube is filtered before it reaches the patient. This filtration protects the patient by removing some of the low-energy photons that are destined to be absorbed by the patient, rather than transferred to the image receptor. In this case, filtration is intended to protect the patient from unnecessary low energy radiation.

RADIATION QUANTITIES AND UNITS

There are several quantities that are used to describe *radiation exposure* and *radiation dose*, including absorbed dose, equivalent dose, and effective dose. These quantities and their associated units will be reviewed in Chapter 9.

Bibliography

1. Bushberg, J.T., Seibert, J.A., Leidholdt, E.M. Jr., and Boone, J.M. (2012). *The Essential Physics of Medical Imaging*. Philadelphia: Wolters Kluwer | Lippincott Williams & Wilkins.
2. Bushong, S. (2017). *Radiologic Science for Technologists*, 11e. Philadelphia: Elsevier.
3. Huda, W. and Slone, R. (2016). *Review of Radiologic Physics*. Philadelphia: Wolters Kluwer.
4. Seeram, E. (2016). *Computed Tomography: Physical Principles, Clinical Applications, and Quality Control*. St Louis, MO: Elsevier.
5. Seeram, E. and Brennan, P. (2017). *Radiation Protection in Diagnostic X-Ray Imaging*. Burlington, MA: Jones and Bartlett Learning.
6. Wolbarst, A.B. (2005). *Physics of Radiology*, 2e. Madison, WI: Medical Physics Publishing.
7. Wolbarst, A.B., Capasso, P., and Wyant, A. (2013). *Medical Imaging: Essentials for Physicians*. Hoboken NJ: Wiley.

4

X-ray tubes and generators

Chapter 3 reviewed the essential physics of all diagnostic x-ray imaging modalities in terms of creating images and paying attention to the dose factors relating to the patient. The relevant physics concepts include the structure of the atom, the nature of radiation, x-ray generation and production, x-ray emission, attenuation of radiation, and the interaction of x-ray with matter.

The purpose of this chapter is to briefly identify and explain how x-rays are generated by presenting a description of the structure and function of the x-ray tube, a topic of vital importance

A Comprehensive Guide to Radiographic Sciences and Technology, First Edition. Euclid Seeram.
© 2021 John Wiley & Sons Ltd. Published 2021 by John Wiley & Sons Ltd.

to the technologist, since the x-ray beam characteristics affect image quality such as image noise, and in particular patient dose. Furthermore, the functional characteristics of three parts of the circuit will be highlighted: the x-ray control console circuit located in the low-voltage section of the circuit, the high-voltage section, and the x-ray tube. Specifically, the elements of the current generation of x-ray generators, the high-frequency generator will be described, and will be followed by a summary of the power rating of the generator. An understanding of the generator will provide the technologist with the tools needed to select and control not only the x-ray beam quality and quantity but also the exposure time appropriate to the nature of the examination.

PHYSICAL COMPONENTS OF THE X-RAY MACHINE

The physical components of the x-ray machine are illustrated in Figure 4.1 which shows a number of components used to produce a beam of radiation from the x-ray tube that is used to produce an image of the patient to be used for diagnostic interpretation. These major components consist of the x-ray control console, the x-ray generator, the x-ray tube, a filter attached to the tube, a collimator, patient, table top, scattered radiation grid, and finally the image detector. These components can be placed into three sections, namely, the console, the generator, and the x-ray tube.

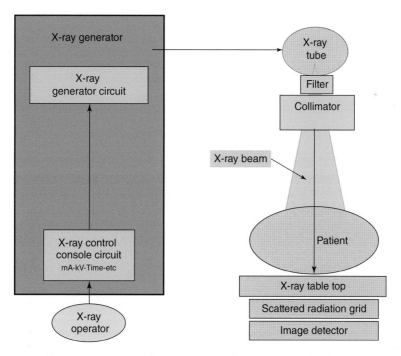

Figure 4.1   The physical components of the x-ray machine. See text for further explanation.

COMPONENTS OF THE X-RAY CIRCUIT

All of these components are connected through an electrical circuit referred to as the *x-ray generator* shown in Figure 4.2. As is clearly illustrated, the major functions of the generator are: (i) to increase the low voltage (volts [v]) from the power company to a high voltage (kilovolts [kV]) which the x-ray tube requires in order to produce x-rays, (ii) to decrease the high current (amperes [A]) from the power company to low current (milliamperes [mA]) needed to control the quantity of x-ray produced, (iii) to convert the alternating current (AC) from the power company to direct current (DC) needed for efficient production of x-rays from the x-ray tube, through a process referred to as rectification, and (iv) to allow the technologist to have full control of technical factors such as the kV, mA, and the exposure time needed for the radiographic examination.

In Figure 4.3, an electrical circuit diagram of the x-ray machine is illustrated. The following are noteworthy:

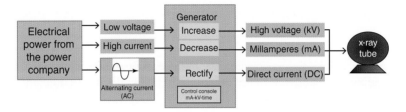

Figure 4.2   The major components of the x-ray generator. See text for further explanation.

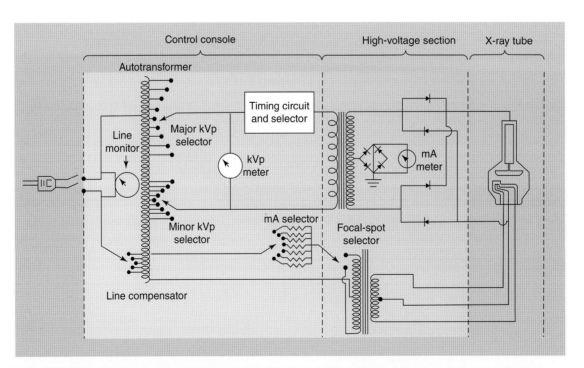

Figure 4.3   An electrical circuit diagram of the x-ray machine. The circuit is divided into three sections: the *control console* (*low-voltage section*), the *high-voltage section*, and the *x-ray tube* which is located in the high-voltage section. Major electrical devices are also shown in each of the low- and high-voltage sections. *Source*: From Bushong [1]. Reproduced by permission.

1. This circuit is divided into three sections, the *control console (low-voltage section)*, the *high-voltage section*, and the *x-ray tube* which is located in the high-voltage section.
2. Major electrical devices in the *low-voltage section* include the autotransformer, kV selection circuits, kV meter, the timer circuit and its selector, and the mA selector.
3. Major electrical devices in the *high-voltage section* include the high-voltage transformer and rectifiers (not labeled and coupled to the x-ray tube), mA meter, focal spot selector (coupled to the x-ray tube), and the x-ray tube itself.
4. The circuit also includes an important feature referred to as the power supply to the generator.

Each of these will now be reviewed in a comprehensive manner as follows:

The power supply to the x-ray circuit

The power supply to the x-ray circuit from the electrical utility company is *AC* with a frequency of 60 cycles per second or 60 Hertz (Hz), in North America and 50 cycles per second or 50 Hz in the United Kingdom and many parts of Europe. The power supply is characterized by the following:

- 1 Hz = 1 cycle per second
- 60 Hz = 60 cycles per second (low frequency)
- 1 cycle per second = 2 impulses per second
- 60 cycles per second = 120 (60 × 2) impulses per second

Furthermore, the AC power can be classified as *single-phase AC power* and *three-phase AC power*. The main features of each of these include:

- *Single-phase AC power.* This power supply is produced by a single-phase AC generator from the utility company and has a single circuit. The circuit produces an AC waveform and has a positive half cycle and a negative half cycle. X-rays are produced only during the positive half cycle, and therefore it is necessary to suppress the negative half cycle during the production of x-rays. Such suppression places the negative half cycle to the positive half of the waveform. X-rays produced by a single-phase x-ray generator are low energy and do not meet the requirements of more sophisticated x-ray examinations requiring more penetrating x-rays and shorter exposure times. Smaller low-powered portable may operate with single-phase power.
- *Three-phase AC power.* A three-phase power supply from the utility company has three separate AC input lines producing three separate waveforms that have the same frequency and voltage amplitude. Rather than being in-phase with each other, however, they are out of phase by one-third of a cycle or by 120°. X-ray production using a three-phase generator is substantially more efficient compared with a single-phase generator. Greater tube output and shorter exposure times are possible.

The low-voltage section (control console)

The following basic components are found on the primary or low-voltage circuit of generator circuit (Figure 4.3):

- *On–off switch.* This switch allows the operator to turn the machine on before imaging the patient and off after use.
- *Line voltage compensator.* Automatic voltage compensation ensures that the correct input voltage is available to the entire circuit in the event of power variations in the hospital. The

incorrect line or supply voltage can affect the output beam from the x-ray tube and, consequently, can have an effect on image quality. The line voltage compensator ensures that the machine receives precisely 220 V (Figure 4.3).

- *Autotransformer*. The input line voltage is delivered to an autotransformer that consists of a single electrical winding to provide the appropriate voltage to the high-voltage circuit, including the filament transformer. The autotransformer not only has primary connections to accommodate the input power (shown on the left side of Figure 4.3) but also secondary connections (on the right side of Figure 4.3) to provide the required voltage to other parts of the circuit. The autotransformer increases the input voltage and also decreases the voltage as well. It works on the principle of electromagnetic induction and is based on the following law referred to as the autotransformer law:

$$\frac{\text{Secondary voltage, } V_s}{\text{Primary voltage, } V_p} = \frac{\text{Number of secondary windings, } N_s}{\text{Number of primary windings, } N_p}.$$

- *kV selector and meter*. The kV is an exposure factor that affects the penetrating power of the beam and can be selected in large (major) or small (minor) increments. The selector is connected to the autotransformer (Figure 4.3). The voltage selected at this point by the technologist is the input voltage to the high-voltage transformer. The kV meter, conversely, is a prereading voltmeter, and because it is positioned across the autotransformer lines, it measures the voltage and not the kV to the x-ray tube. On the control console, however, the kV meter shows the kV that will be applied to the x-ray tube.

- *Filament circuit*. This circuit consists of the filament transformer, mA selector, and the focal spot selector. The circuit determines the filament current (approximately 3–6 A), which affects the tube mA. The mA is the main controlling factor for the quantity of photons from the x-ray tube and is controlled by the filament circuit. The autotransformer provides the voltage to the filament circuit through precision resistors (mA selector). "The filament transformer is a step-down transformer; therefore, the voltage supplied to the filaments is lower, by a factor equal to the turns ratio, than the voltage supplied to the filament transformer. Similarly, the current is increased across the filament transformer in proportion to the turns-ratio" [1]. The focal spot selector allows the technologist to select either a large or small focal spot size appropriate to the requirements of the examination.

- *Exposure timer*. Exposure timer is a manual or automatic electronic timer that determines the length of the exposure (beam-on time) in seconds (s). The product of mA and (s) is the mAs, which is also a controlling factor for the quantity of photons from the x-ray tube.

The high-voltage section

The secondary side of the generator circuit is also called the high-voltage side of the generator. As shown in Figure 4.3, the high-voltage side consists of the high-voltage transformer, rectifiers, the filament transformer, and the mA meter. The high-voltage generator (tank) contains the high-voltage transformer, rectifiers, and the filament transformer, all immersed in oil, which provides electrical insulation.

- *High-voltage transformer*. Because of the turns-ratio (ratio of the number of secondary windings to primary windings), this step-up transformer increases the low-voltage (volts) input from the autotransformer to high voltage (kVs) required for x-ray production. If the turns ratio is 500 : 1 to 1000 : 1, then the input voltage can be increased by approximately 500–1000 times. The input (low voltage) to the high-voltage transformer is AC because transformers operate with AC. The output voltage waveform (high voltage) is also AC, but with greater amplitude than the input waveform.

- *Rectifiers.* Arranged systematically in a circuit called the *rectifier circuit*, rectifiers convert the AC from the high-voltage transformer into *DC* because the x-ray tube requires DC for x-ray production. Modern rectifiers are solid-state, semiconducting materials, such as pure silicon, designed to allow electrons to flow only in one direction. In the x-ray tube, electrons must flow from the cathode to anode, and rectification is responsible for this task. Additionally, rectification can be either *half wave* or *full wave* and the circuit that performs this is a bridge rectifier circuit which shows how the rectifiers are arranged to ensure that electron flow is always from the cathode to anode of the x-ray tube, independent of the high-voltage transformer polarity. *Half-wave rectification* is no longer used in modern radiology departments because this type of circuit uses only the positive half of the AC waveform for x-ray production. The negative half of the AC waveform is not used and is therefore wasted. X-rays are produced in pulses for a total of 60 pulses per second. Therefore, x-ray output is limited with half-wave rectifier circuitry. On the other hand, *full-wave rectification* overcomes this limitation by using the negative half of the AC waveform for x-ray production. For example, using four rectifiers can be used to ensure that electron flow through the x-ray tube (for both the positive and negative portions of the AC waveform) is always from the cathode to anode. X-rays are now produced at 120 pulses per second rather than at 60 pulses per second (for half-wave rectification). Full-wave rectified units produce x-rays more efficiently with shorter exposure times.
- *Filament transformer.* This step-down transformer works with relatively low voltage and high current (about 10V and 5A, respectively). The transformer allows the technologist to provide the appropriate power to the x-ray tube filament for electron emission. The filament current (A) determines the temperature of the filament, thus the number of electrons that will be available for bombarding the target of the x-ray tube. When the filament temperature is higher, the number of electrons available and the quantity of x-rays emitted from the tube are greater.
- The *mA meter*, which is located in the secondary circuit and is connected near the electrical ground (center) of the secondary winding of the high-voltage transformer, measures the tube current (mA), which is the flow of electrons across the x-ray tube during the exposure. This ensures electrical safety, and for this reason, the mA/mAs meter can be placed on the control console.

TYPES OF X-RAY GENERATORS

There are several types of x-ray generators based on their design complexity and cost. These generators include the *single-phase generator*, the *three-phase generator*, the *constant potential generator,* and the *high-frequency generator*. These generator types differ in the efficiency with which they produce x-rays. Each generator type produces a characteristic voltage waveform or ripple (to be described subsequently) and x-ray beam spectra (quality and quantity of photons). While the *voltage ripple* is defined as "the difference between the peak voltage and the minimum voltage, divided by the peak voltage and multiplied by 100%" [2]. *X-ray beam spectra* refer to the intensity and effective beam energy. The following points are noteworthy about the voltage ripple:

- A voltage ripple of 100% means that the voltage going to the x-ray tube varies from zero to some maximum value, the peak of the waveform. As a result, x-rays are produced using a wide range of voltages, that is, low to high (peak). It follows that the x-ray intensity varies from low intensity (for low voltages) to high intensity (as the peak voltage is reached). This factor means that the patient absorbs low-energy x-rays because they have insufficient energy to reach the image receptor. It is logical then to produce x-rays at peak voltages, thus the "**p**" (peak) in kV**p**.
- A ripple of 13% means that the voltage to the x-ray tube begins at 87% of the maximum value and never falls below 87% of the maximum value.
- A ripple of 3% means that the voltage to the x-ray tube never falls below 97% of the maximum value. This value results in higher radiation output (beam quality and quantity), less radiation dose to the patient, and the use of shorter exposure times.

Three-phase generators

The goal of designing and building better generators is to reduce the voltage ripple. A generator with the lowest voltage ripple implies that it provides the most efficient way to produce x-rays.

Three-phase generators overcome the limitations of *single-phase generators* by producing voltage waveforms with low ripple.

Two types of three-phase generators are available:

- *Three-phase, six-pulse generator,* which has six rectifiers to produce a voltage waveform with about 13–25% ripple [2]. This generator produces six pulses per 1/60 of a second compared with two pulses for a single-phase generator.
- *Three-phase 12-pulse generator,* which has 12 rectifiers to produce an output waveform with approximately 3–10% ripple [2].

High-frequency generators

X-ray equipment including computed tomography (CT) scanners now use very sophisticated *high-frequency generators*, which are small, compact, and very efficient in producing x-ray beams needed for imaging in CT. A generalized schematic of a high-frequency generator is illustrated in Figure 4.4.

The electrical components of a high-frequency generator are beyond the scope of this text; however, the following points are necessary to understand how these generators work:

- First the *low-voltage, low-frequency current* (60 Hz) from the main power supply is converted to *high-voltage, high-frequency current* as it passes through the components.
- Second, each component changes the low-voltage, low-frequency AC waveform to supply the x-ray tube with high-voltage, high-frequency DC of almost constant potential.
- The third point to note is that after high-voltage rectification and smoothing, the voltage ripple from a high-frequency generator is less than 1%, compared with 4% from a three-phase, 12-pulse generator. This makes the high-frequency generator more efficient at x-ray production than its predecessor. The power ratings allow the operator to use the appropriate *exposure technique factors*.

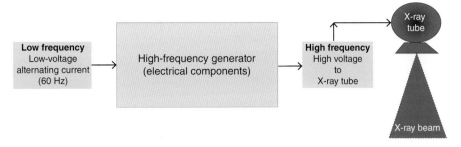

Figure 4.4 A generalized schematic of a high-frequency generator. See text for further details.

Power ratings

The power rating of an x-ray generator takes into consideration the input voltage, the high voltage, and the filament transformer.

- Power = amperes × volts (for constant current and voltage).
- The unit of power is the watt (W).
- The power rating of an x-ray generator is given in kilowatts (kW).
- The benchmark used for x-ray generators is 100 kV and the maximum ampere rating available for a 0.1 second exposure. As given by Bushberg [2], power is expressed algebraically as:

$$\text{Power (kW)} = 100\ \text{kV} \times 1 \left(A_{max} \text{ for a } 0.1 \text{ s exposure} \right).$$

The power requirements for an x-ray generator should be based on the requirements of the particular clinical applications. Additionally, the power rating should be in terms of the focal spot size required for the application. A larger focal spot will have a higher power rating compared with a small focal spot size.

- General radiographic imaging generators commonly have power ratings ranging from 30 to 50 kW for focal spot dimensions of 0.6 mm × 0.6 mm; and lower power ratings of 5–15 kW for smaller focal spots dimensions of 0.3 mm × 0.3 mm^2.
- Angiography and interventional imaging applications generally require generator power ratings of 80–120 kW^2.

THE X-RAY TUBE: STRUCTURE AND FUNCTION

To produce x-rays efficiently and to meet the criteria for optimizing image quality with reduced dose to the patient, an x-ray tube must be designed to provide:

- extremely sharp images (high spatial resolution).
- short exposure times to image moving structures without blurring resulting from motion.
- capability for withstanding large electrical loads (kV, mA, and time) referred to as heat loading.
- proper energy spectrum that is appropriate to the requirements of the examination. For example, a low-kV technique will produce soft x-rays (low energy and less penetrating) required to image soft tissues.
- rapid heat dissipation (cooling).

There are a number of components of the x-ray tube designed specifically to meet the above requirements, and they will be described in section "Major Components."

Major components

The x-ray tube and a small part of the electrical circuit showing the links needed when exposure technique factors (mA and kV) are applied (to the x-ray tube) to produce an x-ray beam are shown in Figure 4.5. The beam intensity (*quantity*) of x-ray photons and the penetrating power (*quality*) are controlled by the mA and the kV, respectively. Two types of x-ray tubes used in radiology are low-powered *stationary anode x-ray tubes* and the more high-powered *rotating anode x-ray tubes*. This chapter will focus on a description of major features of rotating-anode x-ray tubes, since they are widely used in almost all radiographic imaging equipment.

The essential components of an x-ray tube include the cathode assembly, anode assembly, rotor and stator, tube envelope, and x-ray tube housing (Figure 4.5).

- *Cathode Assembly.* The major components of the cathode assembly are a *filament* positioned in a metal cup, called a *focusing cup*. The filament is the source of electrons and is made of tungsten wire wound in a helical coil to increase its surface area. Tungsten is used because of its high melting point (3422 °C), and its high atomic number (Z = 74). Furthermore, the filament is heated via the filament circuit of the generator with approximately 3–6 A to "boil-off" electrons by *thermionic emission*. As the tube ages, the tungsten may vaporize and cause a buildup in the inside of the envelope resulting in electrical arcing during use. Vaporization of the tungsten is the most common cause of tube failure.

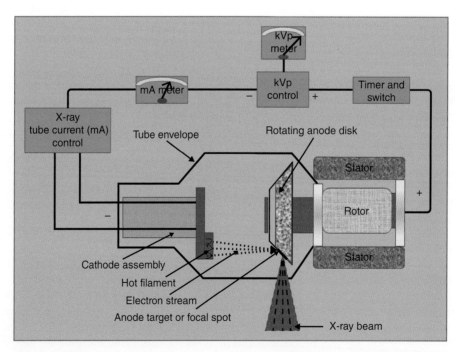

Figure 4.5 The essential components of an x-ray tube include the cathode assembly, anode assembly, rotor and stator, tube envelope, and x-ray tube housing.

To address this problem, tungsten filaments are coated with a layer of thorium (thoriated-tungsten filaments); thus the efficiency of thermionic emission is much greater compared with pure tungsten filaments.

Most x-ray tubes are provided with two filaments positioned in the focusing cup: a *large filament* and a *small filament*. Although the large filament is used for examinations requiring a high-output intensity in a short time (e.g. abdomen, chest), the smaller filament is preferred when detail is important. The focusing cup on the other hand, has a negative charge and plays a role in focusing the electrons from the filament to strike the anode on a region called the target or focal spot. The flow of electrons from the cathode to anode is the tube current or mA. Electrons flow only when there is a potential difference (kV) between the cathode and anode.

- *Anode Assembly.* There are two types of anodes: stationary and rotating. Anodes are characterized by several elements that play a role in the efficiency of x-ray production, image quality, heat loading, and heat dissipation (cooling).

A stationary anode is made of a copper block in which a rectangular piece of tungsten is embedded. The tungsten is the *target*. The copper block conducts heat away from the tungsten target. Additionally, the face of the anode is inclined at an angle, called the *target angle*, to direct the radiation beam to the patient. Inclining the anode at specified angles leads to a design referred to as the *line focus principle*. This principle ensures a large area for heating and a small effective focal spot size. The effective focal spot is the focal spot projected onto the image receptor. When the target angle is small, the effective focal spot size is also small, and the spatial resolution (detail) of the image is better. X-ray tubes have target angles ranging from 5° to 15°. As the target angle is increased, the field coverage at the image receptor is greater. Larger focal spot sizes can withstand greater electrical loads (kV, mA, and time in seconds [mAs]) and have higher heat capacities compared with smaller focal spots. For example, higher mA and short exposure times can be safely used with large focal spots.

The line focus principle gives rise to the heel effect, during which the x-ray beam intensity along the anode–cathode axis varies. The relative intensity is 100% at the cathode side and decreases to approximately 50% at the anode side. This variation in intensity is a result of the fact that because x-rays are produced inside the target, the x-rays leaving the target at the anode side have to travel a longer distance through the target and are therefore absorbed, lowering the intensity at the anode side.

Stationary anode tubes are limited in their x-ray output (intensity) and heat loading. These tubes are suitable for applications that require only a low x-ray output, such as dental radiography and portable fluoroscopy. These limitations are overcome by the rotating anode x-ray tubes.

The rotating anode is a disk supported by a molybdenum stem (Figure 4.5). The basic features of the disk are as follows:

- The diameter of the disk affects the maximum permissible electrical load (kVp, mAs) that the tube can withstand. The diameter varies and can range from 50 to 200 mm. The larger diameter increases the exposure technique factors that the tube can withstand. Because the electron beam strikes a larger target area, the heat capacity of the tube increases.
- Earlier tubes used a pure tungsten disk. However, current state-of-the-art x-ray tubes use a *compound anode disk*. The compound anode disk is made of two or more metals and consists of a base body onto which a coating layer (layer bombarded by the electron beam) is deposited. These materials include rhenium (R), zirconium (Z), and titanium (T) used in conjunction with tungsten (T), molybdenum (M), and graphite. A typical compound anode is the rhenium–tungsten–molybdenum (RTM) disk with molybdenum and/or graphite as the

base, with 10% rhenium and 90% tungsten (coating layer). Compound anode disks have several advantages compared with pure tungsten disks.

- ○ Lesser rotational problems because of the lighter weight.
- ○ Extreme resistance to the aging process.
- ○ Greater heat storage capacity.
- ○ Less roughening of the target track.
- ○ A high and uniform dose over the entire life of the tube.
- ○ Higher exposure technique factors (with shorter exposure times) can be used.

- Target materials for x-ray tubes should have a high atomic number (Z), high thermal conductivity, and high melting point. The efficiency of x-ray production is directly proportional to Z. Higher Z materials produce x-rays more efficiently compared with lower Z materials.

- Rotating anode disks also feature two focal spot sizes (large and small) and have target angles that vary from 5° to 15°. In addition, these anodes are also subject to the anode heel effect.

- An induction motor that consists of a stator and a rotor produces the rotation of the anode disk (Figure 4.5). The purpose of rotating the disk is to increase the instantaneous heat load on the target (thereby increasing the x-ray output by increasing the effective surface area of the target). The induction motor produces the rotation speed of the disk and depends on the frequency of main supply to the stator. Typical speeds are approximately 3600 revolutions per minute (rpm). Increasing the rotation speed increases the heat capacity of the tube. Tubes with high-speed anode rotation rotate at 10 000 rpm. The induction motor consists of the stator that contains electrical windings to provide the force for anode rotation and the rotor.

- Free and smooth rotation of the disk are made possible through the use of steel ball bearings lubricated with metallic barium, silver, or lead; ordinary lubricants reduce friction in the rotor assembly. Ball-bearing technology may result in mechanical problems from heating and cooling. To overcome this problem, a liquid-bearing method is now used in current state-of-the-art, high-capacity x-ray tubes, especially x-ray tubes used in CT [3]. With liquid-bearing technology, the fixed shaft of the anode consists of grooves that contain gallium-based, liquid metal alloy. During anode rotation, the liquid is forced into the grooves, which causes a hydroplaning effect between the sleeve and the liquid. This technology conducts heat away from the disk more efficiently than ball-bearing technology. Additionally, the liquid-bearing technology is free of noise and vibrations.

- "When the operator pushes the exposure button of the radiographic unit, there is a one second wait before taking an exposure. This allows the rotor to accelerate to its designed revolutions per minute. During this time, filament current is increased to provide the correct x-ray tube current. When using a two-position exposure switch, it is important for the radiographer to push the switch to its final position in one motion. That minimizes the time that the filament is heated, which prevents excessive space charge and thus prolongs tube life" [1].

- *X-ray tube envelope and housing*

The x-ray tube *envelope* (also referred to as the *tube insert*) of an x-ray tube is an important component that serves several functions such as supporting the internal components (anode and cathode structures) of the tube; maintaining a vacuum (any gas molecules in the tube will impede the flow of electrons from the cathode to anode. The gas may also cause oxidization of the filament and result in tube failure).

All tube envelopes have an *exit window or port* (through which x-rays leave the tube) that is thinner than the envelope itself. This port filters the beam (inherent filtration) as it exits the tube.

X-ray tube envelopes can be *glass*, *glass and metal*, or completely *metal*. High-capacity x-ray tubes have full metal envelopes. The problems with glass envelopes are limited heat storage capacity and less efficient heat dissipation, because metal deposits seriously affect the physical properties of glass. These problems are overcome with metal envelopes. Recent x-ray tubes have been designed with glass and metal envelopes and with full metal envelopes. The glass and metal envelope tube is a rotating anode xray tube having the same features described earlier, with a few notable differences.

1. The envelope consists of two glass end pieces with a central metal envelope.
2. The metal envelope encases the electric field between the cathode and anode and is not affected by tungsten deposits, compared with glass envelopes.
3. Higher tube currents and shorter exposure times can be used.
4. Two windows are provided: a beryllium window followed by an aluminum window.
5. A large-volume anode disk is a characteristic feature of the glass and metal x-ray tube. The size of this disk allows the technologist to use higher exposure technique factors (with shorter exposure times), increases heat storage capacity, and allows for more efficient heat dissipation.

The envelope of the x-ray tube is encased in a protective housing called the *tube housing or tube shield*. The housing is cylindrical in shape and has two receptacles to accommodate the high-voltage cables from the generator. The purpose of the tube housing is to provide mechanical support for the insert, radiation shielding (ray-proofing), and electrical insulation. Oil is placed between the envelope and the inner walls of the housing to insulate and protect the housing from the high voltage applied to the tube and to facilitate heat dissipation. The housing is lined internally with thin sheets of lead to prevent radiation from "leaking" through the housing (ray-proofing). The protection guidelines for the housing require that the housing must reduce the leakage radiation to less than $26\,\mu C/kg$ – hour ($100\,mR/hr$), $1\,m$ from the x-ray tube [1].

SPECIAL X-RAY TUBES: BASIC DESIGN FEATURES

One significant design feature of x-ray tubes specifically for increasing the heat loading capacity of the x-ray tube is the *metal-ceramic tube with double bearings* design. The most important features in the design of this tube are the metal envelope, ceramic insulation, double-bearing axle, and the large anode disk.

The *metal envelope* ensures higher capacity, better mechanical stability, and better thermal and electrical properties than glass, making it suitable for use in angiography. Furthermore, the metal envelope is not susceptible to metal deposits from vaporization. Additionally, the tube exit window features both beryllium and an interchangeable aluminum filter that can be changed to suit the requirements of the examination. Oil is also used to provide inherent filtration and electrical insulation.

Ceramic is bonded at both ends (cathode and anode) of the tube to ensure a tight vacuum seal as well as to insulate the tube for voltages up to $150\,kV$. Ceramic is also used at the rotor end of the anode and rotates with it and provides insulation of the disk and axle at high voltages.

Double-bearing axle

Conventional tubes have single-bearing axles to support the anode disk. The metal-ceramic tube, by virtue of its construction, can facilitate a larger disk than its counterparts. The disk is mounted onto a double-bearing axle. The purpose of this design is to ensure that the bearing load is more uniform (compared with conventional tubes). The disk for this type of tube is extremely large, approximately 200 mm in diameter. Larger disks provide improved cooling and the use of higher exposure technique factors (with shorter exposure times) compared with conventional tubes.

HEAT CAPACITY AND HEAT DISSIPATION CONSIDERATIONS

When high-speed electrons strike the target, about 1% of the energy supplied to the tube is converted into x-rays and 99% is converted into heat. The x-ray tube must be capable of handling this heat efficiently so that more exposures can be applied to the tube. Understanding x-ray tube heat capacity warrants a brief description of heat loading, heat units (HU), x-ray tube rating, and heat dissipation. These topics are important to the technologist since they play a vital role in preventing tube failure, thus extending the life of the x-ray tube.

The *heat loading* of an x-ray tube is defined as the amount of heat deposited during the application of one exposure. The *HU*, on the other hand, is used to quantify the heat loading of an x-ray tube. A heat unit is the product of mA, kV, exposure time, and a constant that depends on the type of generator (voltage waveform) used. The application of 1 mA, 1 kV for one second will produce 1 HU in the tube (for single-phase generators). For three-phase or high-frequency generators, a multiplicative factor of 1.35 is used "because of their lower voltage ripple and higher average voltage" [2]. For fluoroscopy, the HU/s is equal to the kV × mA. HUs relate to the *heat storage capacity* of the tube. During operation of the x-ray tube, it is important to dissipate the heat produced so that the tube can be operated continuously and one does not have to wait for the tube to cool before another exposure can be applied.

There are three processes by which heat is dissipated in the xray tube: conduction, convection, and radiation. Heat is transferred from the focal track to the anode body by conduction (energy transfer from one region to the next region of the object) and by radiation (emission of the infrared radiation) from the focal track to the tube housing. Heat is transferred from the anode body to the tube housing by radiation. Heat is transferred from the tube housing to the atmosphere in the room by convection.

X-RAY BEAM FILTRATION AND COLLIMATION

As described in Chapter 3, the x-ray beam from the x-ray tube is a heterogeneous beam of radiation, as opposed to a homogeneous beam (Chapter 3). While a homogeneous beam consists of photons that have the same energy (same wavelength), a heterogeneous beam consists of photons that have different energies; that is, the beam is made up of long and short wavelength x-rays. These long wavelength x-rays are low-energy x-rays that have insufficient energy to penetrate the patient to reach the film and are therefore absorbed by the patient. This absorption results in an unnecessary increase in patient dose. It makes good sense then that if these low-energy x-rays can be selectively removed from the beam, then the dose to the patient would be reduced. To accomplish this goal, a filter is used.

The x-ray tube *filter* can be any of the following materials such as aluminum (Al), copper, and tin that absorb, preferentially, low-energy rays from the x-ray beam, and this process is referred to as *filtration*. Al is used mainly since it removes low-energy x-ray photons efficiently. Additionally, *heavy elements* such as gadolinium, iron, samarium, holmium, and tungsten have been used as filter materials in radiographic imaging, particularly in pediatric imaging. These filters play a significant role in skin dose reduction because they provide more attenuation compared with aluminum. In summary, filtration reduces patient dose and is required in any x-ray procedure. The filter is located near the x-ray tube and is always positioned between the tube and the patient.

Inherent and added filtration

There are two types of filtration, namely, inherent filtration and added filtration. *Inherent filtration* is due to the glass or metal envelope, the oil in the tube housing, the exit window of the tube, and cannot be changed, and is generally 0.5 mm aluminum equivalent; however, x-ray tubes designed for mammography occasionally have *beryllium* rather than glass as their exit window providing an inherent filtration of approximately 0.1 mm aluminum equivalent. Inherent filtration cannot be changed by the technologist. As the x-ray tube ages, tungsten may be deposited on the inside of the glass envelope resulting from vaporization of the tungsten filament. This buildup of tungsten deposit will increase the inherent filtration. *Added filtration* on the other hand includes the use of a sheet of aluminum close to the exit window of the x-ray tube. This point is also where the collimator is attached to the x-ray tube. The technologist has control of the amount of added filtration based on the kilovolts peak (kV) used for the examination. Furthermore, the type and thickness of the added filter depends on the kV being used. The higher the kV, the thicker the filter.

The *total filtration* for radiographic imaging system is equal to the inherent filtration + added filtration + filtration by the mirror of the collimator. Radiation Protection regulations and guidelines require that the total permanent filtration must be as follows [4]:

- 0.5 mm aluminum equivalent below 50 kV.
- 1.5 mm aluminum equivalent for voltages between 50 and 70 kV.
- 2.5 mm aluminum equivalent for voltages above 70 kV.

Effects of filtration on x-ray tube output intensity

As reviewed in Chapter 3, the x-ray tube output intensity can be described in terms of x-ray quantity and x-ray quality. While *x-ray quantity* is the number of x-ray photons in the beam of radiation emerging from the x-ray tube, *x-ray quality* refers to the penetrating power or energy of the photons. Filtration reduces the beam quantity and increases beam quality because low-energy photons are selectively removed by the filter. As filtration increases, beam quantity decreases and beam quality (the mean energy of the photons) increases. This factor explains why filtration reduces patient dose and protects the patient from unnecessary radiation. The increase in the mean or effective energy of the beam is referred to as beam hardening.

Half-value layer

The half-value layer (HVL) is used to measure x-ray beam quality. It is defined as the thickness of any absorbing material (filter) needed to reduce the beam intensity to one-half of its original intensity. As noted by Bushong [1], "a diagnostic x-ray beam usually has an HVL in the range of 3–5 mm Al or 3–6 cm of soft tissue" and the HVL "is the best method for specifying x-ray quality."

Collimation

The collimator or any other beam restrictor controls the size of the x-ray beam directed to the patient and the image receptor. Beam-restricting devices include cones, cylinders, variable-aperture collimators, diaphragms, and extension cylinders. Among these devices, the variable-aperture collimator is the most popular because it can shape the field size by moving pairs of lead leaves to produce square or rectangular field sizes. This action is referred to as *collimation*. *Positive beam limitation* (PBL) refers to automatic field collimation. A PBL system ensures that the primary beam is collimated automatically to the size of the image receptor placed in the Bucky tray.

In an effort to improve image contrast from scatter degradation influenced by the x-ray beam field size, the smallest possible field size must be used for body part under examination; that is, collimate the beam to the size of the image receptor or smaller. The International Commission on Radiological Protection (ICRP) states that, in terms of the factors affecting the dose to the patient, the most significant is limiting the xray field size to the anatomic area of interest. Collimation reduces the genetically significant dose (GSD = the population gonadal dose) by 65% [1].

References

1. Bushong, S. (2017). *Radiologic Science for Technologists. Physics, Biology, and Protection*, 11e. St Louis: Elsevier.
2. Bushberg, J.T., Seibert, J.A., Leidholdt, E.M. Jr., and Boone, J.M. (2012). *The Essential Physics of Medical Imaging*, 3e. Philadelphia: Wolters Kluwer/Lippincott Williams & Wilkins.
3. Seeram, E. *Computed Tomography: Physical Principles, Clinical Applications, and Quality Control*, 4e. St Louis, MO: Elsevier.
4. National Council on Radiation Protection and Measurements (NCRP) (1989). *Medical X-Ray, Electron Beam and Gamma Ray Protection for Energies up to 50 MeV: Equipment Design, Performance and Use* (Report 102) NCRP, Bethesda, MD.

5

Digital image processing at a glance

A characteristic feature of digital radiographic imaging systems used in diagnostic radiology such as digital radiography (DR) including computed radiography (CR) and flat-panel digital radiography (FPDR); digital fluoroscopy (DF); digital mammography (DM); digital radiographic tomosynthesis (DRT) and digital breast tomosynthesis (DBT) is digital image processing. In this chapter, the general concepts of digital image processing which can be applied to the images produced by each of these modalities, and which are commonplace in clinical practice, will be highlighted.

DIGITAL IMAGE PROCESSING

Digital image processing has become commonplace in a DR environment [1]. Images displayed on display monitors can be manipulated to meet the needs of the observer. Image processing is intended to enhance the visual task of interpretation of images, and the assessment of what constitutes an image of diagnostic quality. For example, while the visual task of a radiologist is lesion detection, the viewing task of the technologist on the other hand is to assess the quality of the displayed image that characterizes a diagnostic quality image.

A Comprehensive Guide to Radiographic Sciences and Technology, First Edition. Euclid Seeram.
© 2021 John Wiley & Sons Ltd. Published 2021 by John Wiley & Sons Ltd.

Definition

Digital image processing is defined as processing of images using a digital computer, and the result of computer processing is a *digital image*, displayed on a monitor for viewing and interpretation.

Image formation and representation

Digital image processing requires an understanding of the general nature of images, and as such Castleman [2] conceptualizes images as a subset of all objects and that the image set contain subsets, such as visible images, non-visible images, optical images, and mathematical images. Visible images, for example, include photographs, drawings, and paintings. Non-visible images on the other hand include temperature, pressure, and elevation maps. Optical images are holograms, for example. Finally, mathematical images include continuous and discrete functions, as is clearly illustrated in Figure 5.1, and these functions can be used to create two categories of images used in radiology namely, an analog image and a digital image (Figure 5.1).

In DR, x-rays transmitted through the patient falls upon a detector which converts the attenuated x-rays into a continuous signal called an analog signal. In a DR imaging system, analog signals must be converted into digital signal (discrete data) using an analog-to-digital converter (ADC). Subsequently, this digital data represent a digital image (Figure 5.2) which must be converted back into an analog image to be displayed on a viewing monitor. This image can be processed using a number of *processing operations* that are meant to enhance diagnostic interpretation.

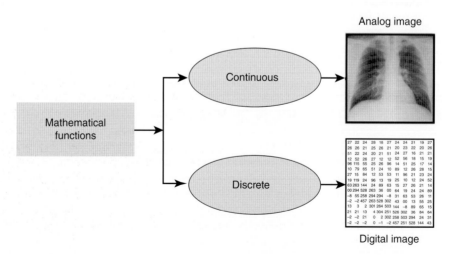

Figure 5.1 Mathematical images include continuous and discrete functions. These functions can be used to create two categories of images used in radiology namely, an analog image and a digital image.

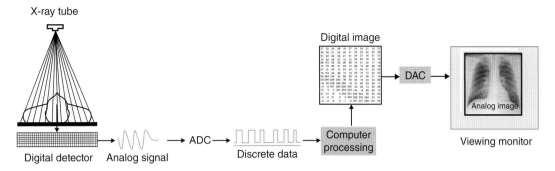

Figure 5.2   In a digital radiography imaging system, analog signals must be converted into digital signal (discrete data) using an analog-to-digital converter (ADC). Subsequently, this digital data represent a digital image which must be converted back into an analog image to be displayed on a viewing monitor.

Processing operations

Processing operations include algorithms [2–5] developed to alter the appearance of image such as point processing operations such as *gray scale processing* (windowing, image subtraction, and temporal averaging), local processing operations (such as spatial filtering, edge enhancement, and smoothing), and global operations such as the Fourier transform (FT). The details of these operations will not be described in this book, and students should refer to Refs. [2–5] for the details of these processing operations. It is important to note that these operations are intended to change the intensity values of the pixels in the input image and display the resulting changes in the output image with the goal of changing the characteristics of the image to suit the viewing needs of the observer in order to enhance diagnosis.

For CR and FPDR, common operations include partitioned pattern recognition, exposure field recognition, histogram analysis, normalization of raw image data, gray scale processing, spatial filtering, dynamic range control, and energy subtraction, for example. Examples of operations used in digital subtracting angiography (DSA) and DF include analytic processing, subtraction of images out of a sequence, gray scale processing, temporal frame averaging, edge enhancement, and pixel shifting. Examples of processing operation in CT include image reformatting, gray scale processing, region of interest, magnification, surface and volume rendering, and so on. It is interesting to note that gray scale processing is common to all of the modalities mentioned above. *Gray scale processing* is called *windowing* and since it is the most widely used operation in DR, it will be described in detail later in this chapter.

CHARACTERISTICS OF DIGITAL IMAGES

As mentioned earlier, a *digital image* is a numerical representation of the patient's anatomy. The major characteristics of a digital image include a matrix, pixels, voxels, and the bit depth [5].

- A *matrix* is made up of a two-dimensional array of numbers, consisting of columns (M) and rows (N) as illustrated in Figure 5.3a. The columns and rows define small square regions called *pixels* or picture elements (Figure 5.3a). The *dimension* of the image can be described by M and N. When M = N, the image is square. In general, DR images are rectangular in shape. When imaging

(a)

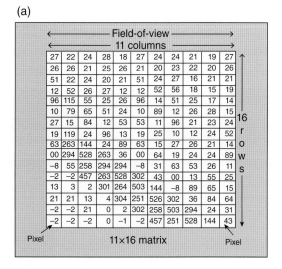

(b)

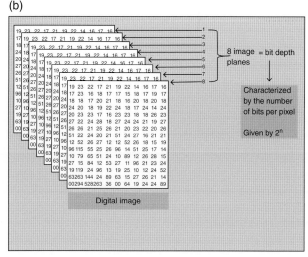

Figure 5.3   The major characteristics of a digital image include a matrix, pixels, voxels, and the bit depth.

patients, technologists select the matrix size typical for the modality and which is sometimes referred to as the *field-of-view* (FOV). Typical matrix sizes for CR, FPDR, DM, DSA, and CT are 2048×2048, 2048×2048, 4096×4096, 1024×1024, and 512×512, respectively.

- The *size* of the image is given by the algebraic expression M×N×k bits, where *k bits* implies that each pixel in the matrix M×N is represented by k binary digits. Since the binary number system uses the base 2, k bits = 2^k.
- The *bit depth* is the number of bits that a pixel can have. Each pixel in the matrix will have 2^k gray levels or density. A digital image with a bit depth of 8 implies that each pixel will have 2^8 (256) gray levels or shades of gray, as shown in Figure 5.3b. Typical bit depths for CR, FPDR, DM, DSA, and CT are 12, 12, 12, 10, and 12, respectively.
- The *size of the pixel* is related to the FOV and the matrix size. This relationship is expressed algebraically as *pixel size = FOV/matrix size*; the larger the matrix size, the smaller the pixel size (for the same FOV) and the better the spatial resolution or sharpness of the image. In a digital image, each pixel value represents information contained in a volume of tissue in the patient. This volume is called a *voxel* (contraction for volume element). Tissue voxel information is converted into numerical values and expressed in the pixels of the image, and these numbers (integers = 0, positive number or a negative number) are assigned brightness levels, as illustrated in Figure 5.4.

GRAY SCALE PROCESSING

There are several classes of digital image processing operations such as point processing operations such as *gray scale processing*, local processing operations (spatial filtering, edge enhancement, and smoothing), and global operations such as the FT. This chapter will only focus on the most common of these operations, gray scale processing, also referred to as *windowing*. The overall goal of image processing is to change the intensity values of the pixels in the input image and display the resulting changes in the output image to suit the needs of the observer. Specifically, image processing is intended to change and optimize image contrast, improve image detail by

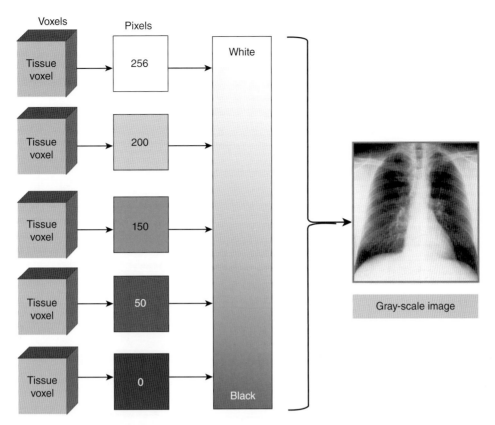

Figure 5.4 Tissue voxel information is converted into numerical values and expressed in the pixels of the image, and these numbers (integers = 0, positive number or a negative number) are assigned brightness levels. This shading is done on purpose to mimic the appearance of structures on a film image, where bone is white and air is black, and where soft tissues are seen as shades of gray.

sharpening the image, and finally decrease the noise present in the image. Windowing is used in CR, DR using flat-panel detectors, DM, DSA, CT, and magnetic resonance imaging (MRI).

Two noteworthy and essential topics of digital image processing are the concepts of the histogram and lookup table (LUT).

- The *histogram* is a graph of the number of pixels in the entire image or part of the image having the same gray levels (density values), plotted as a function of the gray levels, as shown in Figure 5.5.
- The *LUT* uses the input image pixel values and changes them into output pixel values to effect a change in contrast and brightness of the output image, as illustrated in Figure 5.6. "Changing the histogram of the image can alter the brightness and contrast of the image. If the histogram is modified or changed, the brightness and contrast of the image will change as well.
  - This operation is called *histogram modification* or *histogram stretching*. While a wide histogram implies more contrast, a narrow histogram will show less contrast. If the values of the histogram are concentrated in the lower end of the range of values, the image appears dark, as opposed to a bright image, in which case the values are weighted toward the higher end of the range of values" [5].

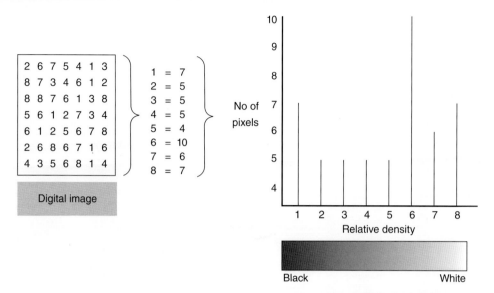

Figure 5.5 The histogram is a graph of the number of pixels in the entire image or part of the image having the same gray levels (density values), plotted as a function of the gray levels.

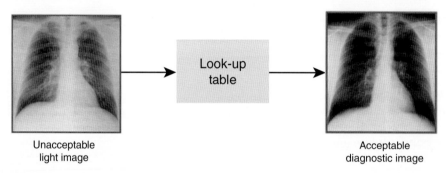

Figure 5.6 The lookup table (LUT) uses the input image pixel values and change them into output pixel values to effect a change in contrast and brightness of the output image.

The LUT is intended to change a poor input image into an acceptable output image to enhance diagnostic interpretation. The LUT determines the numbers assigned to the input pixel values that change them into output pixel values that result in a change in contrast and brightness of the image. Furthermore, the LUT can be represented as a plot of the input image pixel values as a function of the output image pixel values, and the result is a graph that looks like the classic characteristic curve (H and D curve) for film. In review, the slope of the characteristic curve influences the contrast of the image. A steep slope results in a high contrast image while a small slope (less than 45°) will result in decreased contrast. As described by Seeram [5], "digital radiographic imaging systems (CR and DR, for example) utilize a wide range of LUTs stored in the system, for the different types of clinical examinations (chest, spine, pelvis, extremities for example). The operator should therefore select the appropriate LUT to match the part being imaged. An important point to note here is the following: since digital radiographic detectors have wide exposure latitude and a linear response, the image displayed without processing may appear as a low contrast image." A processing example for a chest image using the LUT is shown in Figure 5.6.

Windowing

As noted earlier in this chapter, *windowing* is the most common technique that technologists and radiologists use to change the contrast and brightness of a digital image, as is clearly illustrated in Figure 5.7. Since a digital image is made up of numbers, two important and significant related concepts are in order. These concepts are the *window width* (WW) and the *window level* (WL). While the WW is defined as the range of the numbers in the image (pixel values), the WL is defined as the center of the range of numbers in the image.

In Figure 5.7, while the gray levels represent the range of pixel values in the image, the gray scale is the displayed image contrast. The tissue gray scale is stretched out with white at one end, black at the other, and shades of gray in between. While the lower numbers are assigned dark shades, the higher numbers are assigned light shades. The gray scale changes as the WW is expanded or narrowed. The functions of the WW and WL are to control the image contrast and the image brightness, respectively. In an image, the displayed gray levels will range from $-1/2WW+WL$ to $+1/2WW+WL$. The displayed WW and WL values are always shown on the image. While narrow WW provides improved image contrast, a wide WW will show an image with low contrast, for a WL of 0. This effect is shown in Figure 5.8. On the other hand, when the WL is decreased, the image becomes lighter since more of the higher numbers (assigned light shades) will be displayed in the image as shown in Figure 5.9a for a fixed WW. When the WL is increased, the image appears darker since more of the lower numbers (assigned dark shades) will be displayed in the image as shown in Figure 5.9c for a fixed WW. The acceptable image contrast and brightness are shown in Figure 5.9b.

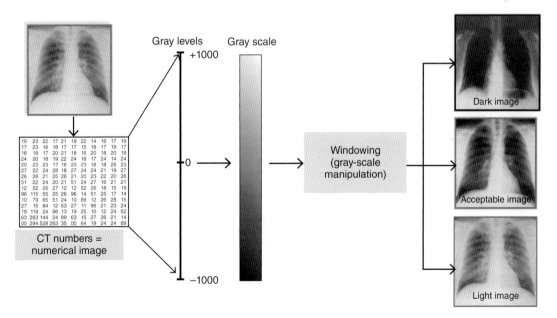

Figure 5.7 Windowing is the most common technique that technologists and radiologists use to change the contrast and brightness of a digital image. While the gray levels represent the range of pixel values in the image, the gray scale is the displayed image contrast. The tissue gray scale is stretched out with white at one end, black at the other, and shades of gray in between. While the lower numbers are assigned dark shades, the higher numbers are assigned light shades. See text for further details.

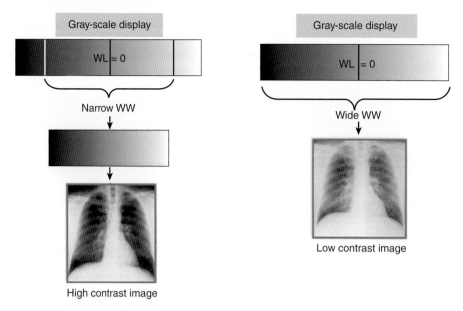

Figure 5.8   The displayed WW and WL values are always shown on the image. While narrow WW provides improved image contrast, a wide WW will show an image with low contrast, for a WL of 0. See text for further explanation.

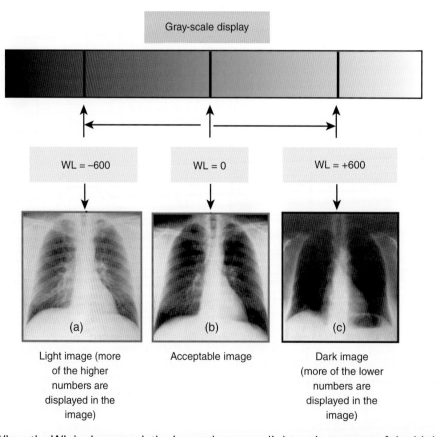

Figure 5.9   When the WL is decreased, the image becomes lighter since more of the higher numbers (assigned light shades) will be displayed in the image as shown in (a) for a fixed WW. When the WL is increased, the image appears darker since more of the lower numbers (assigned dark shades) will be displayed in the image as shown in (c) for a fixed WW. The acceptable image contrast and brightness are shown in (b).

CONCLUSION

As noted by Seeram [5], "image post processing is now a routine activity in digital medical imaging and has become an essential tool in the picture archiving and communication systems (PACS) environment. Already technologists and radiologists are actively involved in using the tools of image processing, such as the digital image processing operations and techniques outlined in this chapter. Education programs for both technologists and radiologists are also beginning to incorporate digital image processing as part of their curriculum. Such activities will only serve to improve communications with radiologists, medical imaging physicists, and biomedical engineers, and with equipment vendors as well."

References

1. Seeram, E. (2004). Digital image processing. *Radiologic Technology* 75 (6): 435–452.
2. Castleman, K.R. (1996). *Digital Image Processing*. Englewood Cliffs, NJ: Prentice Hall.
3. Gonzalez, R.C. and Woods, R.E. (2018). *Digital Image Processing*, 4e. Toronto, ON: Pearson.
4. Solomon, C. and Breckon, T. (2011). *Fundamentals of Digital Image Processing*. West Sussex: Wiley.
5. Seeram, E. (2019). *Digital Radiography: Physical Principles and Quality Control*, 2e. New York, NY: Springer.

6

Digital radiographic imaging modalities: principles and technology

A Comprehensive Guide to Radiographic Sciences and Technology, First Edition. Euclid Seeram.
© 2021 John Wiley & Sons Ltd. Published 2021 by John Wiley & Sons Ltd.

Chapter 2 presented a general overview of the digital radiographic imaging systems used in diagnostic radiology, by identifying and defining briefly the general system components of digital radiography (DR) including computed radiography (CR) and flat-panel digital radiography (FPDR); digital fluoroscopy (DF); digital mammography (DM); digital radiographic tomosynthesis (DRT) and digital breast tomosynthesis (DBT). This chapter will focus on the details of CR, FPDR, and DF, with respect to the essential physical principles and major technical considerations.

COMPUTED RADIOGRAPHY

CR was introduced decades ago replacing film-screen radiography (FSR). Through the years, CR has demonstrated effective use in diagnostic radiography. CR includes two major pieces of equipment: the CR imaging plate (IP) and the CR image processor, sometimes referred to as the CR image reader.

Essential steps

There are four essential steps in the CR imaging process as outlined in Figure 6.1:

1. The IP is exposed to x-rays and captures a latent image of the patient's anatomy under examination.
2. The IP is taken to the image processor to render the latent image visible through digital image processing.
3. The image is displayed for viewing and interpretation.
4. The IP is erased in the image reader to be used again and again.

Basic physical principles

There are two notable physical principles in CR imaging. The first addresses the formation of the latent image, and the second relates to rendering the latent image visible. To understand these two principles, it is important to review the characteristic features of the IP.

The IP consists of a photostimulable storage phosphor (PSP) layered on a base to provide support. Photostimulable phosphors have the property of creating and storing a latent image, when exposed to x-rays. To render the latent image visible, the PSP must be scanned by a laser beam of a specific wavelength. Laser scanning produces a luminescence (light) that is proportional to

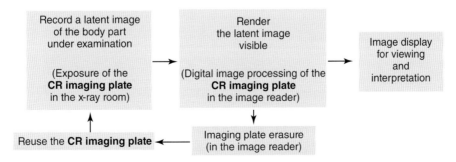

Figure 6.1 Four essential steps in the CR imaging process. See text for further explanation.

the stored latent image. This luminescence is referred to as photostimulable luminescence (PSL). In general, barium fluoro halide: europium (BaFX: Eu^{2+}) meets certain requirements for CR imaging, including good x-ray absorption efficiency; and must be capable of being stimulated by a helium—neon (He—Ne) laser [1]. The halide (X) can be chlorine (Cl), bromine (Br), or iodine (I), or a mixture of them [2]. The phosphor is usually doped with Eu^{2+} which acts as an activator to improve the efficiency of PSL. Another phosphor used in CR is BaFBr/I : Eu^{2+} and recently cesium bromide (CsBr : Eu^{2+}) is now used as a PSP for CR imaging [2].

As described by Seeram [3], "when x-rays fall upon the IP, the europium atoms are ionized by the radiation and the electrons move from the valence band (ground state) to the conduction band (higher energy). Electrons in the conduction band are free to travel to a so-called 'F-center'. F comes from the German and 'Farbe' meaning color [4]. The number of trapped electrons is proportional to the absorbed radiation. It is at the point in the process where the electrons are spatially distributed to create the latent image. In addition to this mechanism, x-ray exposure of the IP causes it to fluoresce (emits light when it is exposed to x-rays) for a very brief duration." After exposure of the IP, it is taken to the image reader for processing.

The IP is scanned in the reader by a laser beam and the laser light must be capable of being absorbed by the "F-centers." This absorption causes the trapped electrons to move up to the conduction band, where they are free to return to the valence band, thus causing the Eu^{3+} to return to the Eu^{2+} state. Transition of the electrons from a higher energy state to a lower energy state (ground state) results in an emission of bluish-purple light (~415 nm wavelength) referred to as PSL. This PSL is very different from the fluorescence described earlier. The lasers used today for PSL in CR units are semiconductor lasers that produce light with a 680 nm wavelength compared to He—Ne lasers that produce light with a 633 nm wavelength used in earlier CR units.

As seen in Figure 6.2, after the latent image is rendered visible (through digital image pre and post processing), it is displayed for viewing and interpretation. At this point, the IP is exposed to a high-intensity light (brighter than the stimulating light) to get rid of any residual

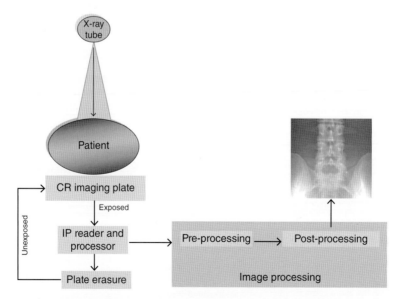

Figure 6.2 This figure shows that after the latent image is rendered visible (through digital image pre and post processing), it is displayed for viewing and interpretation. At this point, the IP is exposed to a high-intensity light (brighter than the stimulating light to get rid of any residual signal left on the IP).

signal left on the IP. The IP is sensitive to background radiation and scattered radiation produced while imaging patients, and in this regard, it must be erased before use, especially if the IP has not been used for a period of time.

Response of the IP to radiation exposure

The response of the x-ray film and the DR detector was briefly described in Chapter 2. This response is important in practice since a good understanding will allow the correct selection of radiographic exposure technique factors for the examination. In summary, the response of film to exposure is described by the characteristic curve or the H and D curve which shows what happens to the film density when the exposures are low (underexposed) and high (overexposed). Low and high exposures result in light and dark film densities, respectively, and render the image useless (Figure 2.2). The slope of the curve defines the useful range of exposures and is referred to as the film latitude or the dynamic range of the film receptor. It also indicates correct exposures resulting in acceptable images. While underexposure results in noisy images, overexposure results in high doses to the patient.

The response of the DR image detector, the IP, is different to that of film and solves the problems identified above imposed by film imaging. The IP has a wide-exposure latitude (Figure 2.3) meaning that the CR IP has a wide dynamic range, a significant advantage of CR. "If the exposure is too low or too high, the image quality is still acceptable due to the ability of the CR system to perform digital image processing to adjust the image quality to match the image quality that would be produced by the optimum exposure. A low exposure (underexposure) will produce high noise (that can be detected by the radiologist), while a high exposure (overexposure) will produce very good images, compared to the optimum image produced by the optimum exposure (appropriate exposure). The problem with high exposures however is related to increased dose to the patient" [3]. Furthermore, Seibert notes that "because of the negative feedback due to underexposures, a predictable and unfortunate use of higher exposures, 'dose creep', is a typical occurrence. To identify an estimate of the exposure used for a given image, CR manufacturers have devised methods to analyze the digital numbers in the image based upon the calibrated response to known incident exposure" [5]. In CR, the technology features a technique referred to as exposure field recognition (EFR) which is intended to provide an indication of the amount of radiation falling upon the CR IP, after it leaves the patient. This is referred to as the *exposure indicator* (EI) or *exposure index*.

DR vendors offer EIs for each of their systems, including several proprietary methods to calculate the EI, which has therefore led to different EI names. For example, although Fuji refers to its indicator as a "sensitivity" (S) number, Carestream uses the term "exposure index" and Agfa uses the term "log of the median of the histogram (lgM)." These differences have created "widespread confusion and frustration" for all those using DR systems [6], and this has provided the motivation for the development of a standardized EI, championed by most notably the International Electrotechnical Commission (IEC) [7] and the AAPM [8].

The standardized exposure indicator

Since the standardized EI is used on all DR systems (DR and FPDR), it is essential to review the major features of this current EI system, established by authoritative groups such as the IEC and the AAPM.

There are several conditions that must be considered:

1. The standardized EI is related to the detector exposure.
2. The standardized EI be obtained from the pixel values in the region of interest.
3. The standardized EI uses a linear proportional scale related to the detector exposure/signal (i.e. doubling the detector dose, doubles the standardized EI value).
4. Other conditions include the radiation beam quality (k, half-value layer, and added filtration) used for the calibration of the EI, and the precision of the scale, expressed as one, two, or more significant digits.

Furthermore, there are four parameters of the IEC standardized EI that are of importance to the technologist, and the radiologist as well. These include the EI, EI_T, DI, and VOI. Each of these will be defined next. The definitions are from the IEC [7] as follows:

- *EI* is a "measure of the detector response to radiation in the relevant image region of an image acquired with a digital x-ray imaging system."
- The *target EI* (EI_T) is the "expected value of the exposure index when exposing the x-ray image receptor properly."
- The *deviation index* (DI) is a "number quantifying the deviation of the actual exposure index from a target exposure index."
- The *volume of interest* (VOI) is the "central tendency of the original data in the relevant image region. The central tendency is a statistical term depicting generally the center of a distribution. It may refer to a variety of measures such as the mean, median, or the mode."

The IEC and the AAPM use common steps to determine the standardized EI, as follows:

- The DR vendor calibrates the detector and produces an EI that is directly proportional to the detector exposure (doubling the exposure doubles the EI value). For example, doubling the dose from 5 to 10 mGy doubles the EI from 500 to 1000, respectively.
- The user (imaging department) establishes an EI_T for each body part, view, and procedure for the detector being used.
- As shown in Figure 6.3, once the image is obtained, the DI is calculated using the following algebraic expression:

$$DI = 10\log_{10}(EI/EI_T).$$

This DI value indicates to the technologist the following information [8]:

- A DI = 0 means that the intended exposure to the detector is correct (i.e. $EI = EI_T$).
- Although a positive DI number indicates overexposure, a negative DI number indicates underexposure.
- A DI number of +1 = an overexposure of 26% more than the desired exposure.
- A DI number of −1 = an underexposure of 20% less than the desired exposure.
- A DI number of +3 = 100% more than the desired exposure.
- A DI number of −3 = 50% less than the desired exposure.
- The acceptable range of DI numbers is approximately +1 to −1, and the DR system is able to deliver the EI_T established by the department.
- Furthermore, numbers greater than +1 and less than −1 would indicate gross overexposure and underexposure, respectively, as shown in Figure 6.4.

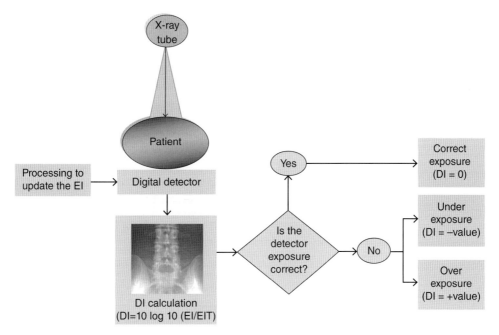

Figure 6.3   The essential steps for calculation of the DI in the new EI paradigm.

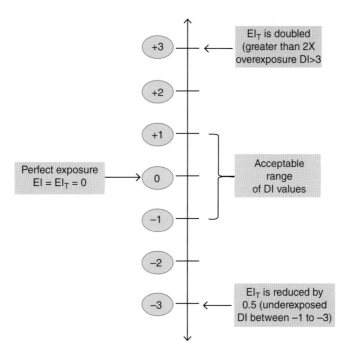

Figure 6.4   The acceptable range of DI numbers is approximately −1 to +1, and the DR system is able to deliver the EIT established by the department. Furthermore, numbers greater than +3 and between −1 and −3 would indicate gross overexposure and underexposure, respectively.

FLAT-PANEL DIGITAL RADIOGRAPHY

The motivation for the development of other DR systems such as FPDR stems from the shortcomings of CR. Compared to FSR, CR offers inefficient detection efficiency, and lower spatial resolution. Furthermore, CR IPs can easily be damaged (when dropped accidently) and are susceptible to cracking and scratches, and must be transported physically to the image processor (image reader) [9].

What is FPDR?

A flat-panel DR imaging system is based on the use of a flat-panel digital detector and thus is considered a single unit (a thin flat-panel device) that consists of a flat-panel x-ray detection array, and the associated electronics (preamplifiers, switching control, the central logic circuits, the analog-to-digital converters [ADCs], and internal memory) as illustrated in Figure 6.5. A noteworthy point about FPDR systems is that x-ray detection and digitization of the x-ray signal take place within the flat-panel detector (FPD).

Types of FPDR systems

Two types of FPDR detectors have become commonplace. These include *indirect detectors* and *direct detectors* based on the type of x-ray absorber. While indirect detectors use a phosphor (Figure 6.6a), direct detectors use a photoconductor, as shown in Figure 6.6b.

Basic physical principles of indirect and direct flat-panel detectors

In Figure 6.6a, the components of the indirect FPD are shown. These include an *x-ray scintillator* (x-ray conversion layer), positioned onto an *amorphous silicon (a-Si) photodiode* flat-panel

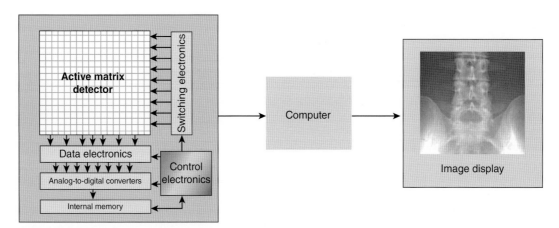

Figure 6.5 A flat-panel DR imaging system is based on the use of a flat-panel digital detector and thus is considered a single unit (a thin flat-panel device) that consists of a flat-panel x-ray detection array, and the associated electronics (preamplifiers, switching control, the central logic circuits, the ADCs, and internal memory).

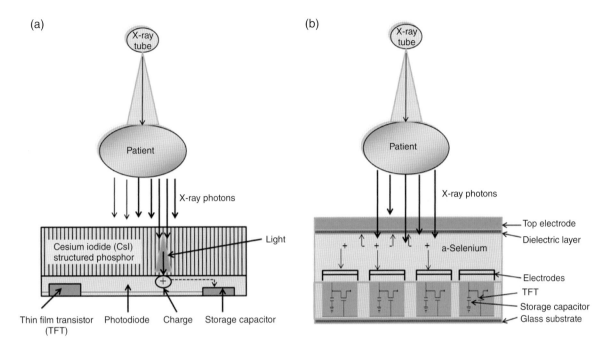

Figure 6.6 Two types of flat-panel digital radiography detectors have become commonplace. These include *indirect detectors* and *direct detectors* based on the type of x-ray absorber. While indirect detectors use a phosphor (a), direct detectors use a photoconductor, as shown in (b).

layer, with a *thin-film transistor* (TFT) array for readout of the electrical charges by the photodiode array. The following are major points to consider:

1. The x-ray scintillator layer is usually *cesium iodide (CsI)* or *gradolinium oxysulfide* (Gd_2O_2S). While CsI crystals are deposited in a needle-like fashion (structured phosphor) and run in the direction of the x-ray beam, Gd_2O_2S crystals are deposited as powdered particles (turbid phosphor). While the former is sometimes referred to as a structured scintillator, the latter is referred to as an unstructured scintillator.

2. Furthermore, powdered phosphors produce lateral spreading of light, which destroys the spatial resolution of the image. Structured phosphors like the CsI needles on the other hand reduce the lateral dispersion of light, thus improving the spatial resolution of the image.

3. The a-Si photodiode layer converts the light from the x-ray detection scintillator into electrical charges. Adjacent to the a-Si photodiode layer is a TFT array, as well as storage capacitors and associated electronics. The capacitor collects and stores the electrical charge produced in the a-Si photodiode array.

Figure 6.6b illustrates the essential components of the direct FPD. Major components include a source of high voltage, top electrode, dielectric layer, photoconductor, collection electrode, TFT, storage capacitor, and the glass substrate. The photoconductor is *amorphous selenium (a-Se)* although other photoconductors such as lead oxide, lead iodide, thallium bromide, and gadolinium compounds can be used [8]. The a-Se provides excellent x-ray photon detection properties and provides images with very high spatial resolution. The photoconductor detects x-ray photons from the patient and converts them directly into electrical charges. The TFT and associated electronics (capacitors for example) collect and store the changes for subsequent readout. The following points are noteworthy about the FPD:

1. The panel design is referred to as an *active matrix array*, consists of rows and columns shown in Figure 6.5.
2. Each pixel contains a TFT (switch), a storage capacitor, and a sensing area, referred to as the sensing/storage element.
3. Apart from the matrix of pixels, there are other electronic components such as switching electronics to activate each row of pixels, and electronic amplifiers and associated electronic devices (multiplexer) for signal readout from each column of pixels.
4. The electronic signal (analog signal) is subsequently sent to the *ADC* for digitization. The ADC is also included in the FPD. Finally, the digital data stream is sent to a digital computer for digital image processing.

The fill factor of the pixel in the flat-panel detector

The *fill factor* of the flat-panel digital detector active matrix array is shown in Figure 6.7. As illustrated, each pixel contains generally three components: the TFT, the capacitor, and the sensing area. The fill factor then is defined as the ratio of sensing area of the pixel to the area of the pixel itself [9], and can be expressed as:

Fill factor = sensing area of the pixel / area of the pixel.

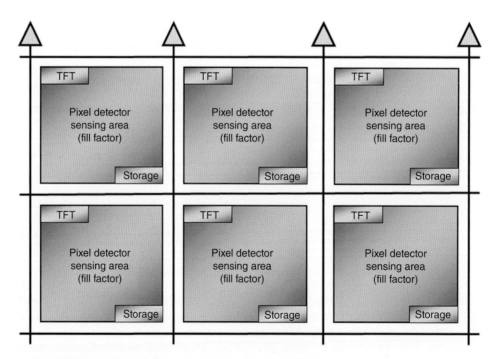

Figure 6.7   The fill factor then is defined as the ratio of sensing area of the pixel to the area of the pixel itself. See text for further details.

The fill factor is also expressed as a percentage, where a fill factor of 80% means that 20% of the pixel area is occupied by the detector electronics with 80% representing the sensing area. The fill factor affects both the spatial resolution (detail) and contrast resolution (signal-to-noise ratio [SNR]) characteristics of the detector [9]. Detectors with high fill factors (large sensing areas) will provide better spatial and contrast resolution than detectors with low fill factors (small sensing area).

Exposure indicator

The *EI* is a useful tool to address the problem of "exposure creep." The EIs for DR systems are based on the concepts of the *standardized EI*.

Image quality descriptors for DR systems

The *image quality descriptors* for DR systems include spatial resolution (detail), density resolution, noise, detective quantum efficiency (DQE), and artifacts. These will be reviewed in some detail in Chapter 7; however, the following description in noteworthy:

- The *spatial resolution* of a digital image is related to the size of the pixels in the image matrix.
- The *density resolution* of a digital image is linked to the *bit depth*, which is the range of gray levels per pixel.
- The *noise* on the other hand can be related to electronic noise (system noise) and *quantum noise (quantum mottle)*. The quantum noise is determined by the number of x-ray photons (the signal, S) falling upon the detector to create the image.
- The *DQE* is a measure of the efficiency and fidelity with which the detector can perform the task of converting an input exposure to a useful output image.
- An *artifact* is "any false visual feature on a medical image that simulates tissue or obscures tissue" [5]. An earlier definition of an artifact is provided by Willis et al. who states that "an artifact is a feature in an image that masks or mimics a clinical feature" [10].

Continuous quality improvement for DR systems

The concept of *continuous quality improvement (CQI)* includes *quality assurance (QA)* and *quality control (QC)* programs that are essential not only for optimizing the assessment and evaluation of patient care, but also for monitoring the performance of equipment. QA and QC will be described in Chapter 8. While QA refers to systems and procedures for assuring quality patient care and deals with the administrative aspects of patient care and quality outcomes, QC refers specifically to the monitoring of important variables that affect image quality and radiation dose, including the technical aspects (rather than administrative aspects) of equipment performance. CQI, QA, and QC are intended to ensure optimum image quality for the purpose of enhancing diagnosis, to reduce the radiation dose to both patients and personnel and to reduce costs to the institution.

In particular, QC includes activities that range from acceptance testing, and routine performance, to error correction [9]. While *acceptance testing* is the first major step in a QC program and it ensures that the equipment meets the specifications set by the manufacturers, *routine performance* involves performing the actual QC test on the equipment with varying degrees of frequency (annually, semiannually, monthly, weekly, or daily). *Error correction* ensures that equipment not meeting the performance criteria or tolerance limit established for specific QC tests must be replaced or repaired to meet tolerance limits.

DIGITAL FLUOROSCOPY

Fluoroscopy is a dynamic imaging modality that shows anatomical structures, the motion of organs, and the movement of contrast media in blood vessels and organs with the goal of obtaining functional information. Fluoroscopy has evolved from what has been referred to as *conventional fluoroscopy* to DF. While the former recorder images i on film (static and dynamic images), DF images are dynamic image recorder and stored in a computer. The term conventional fluoroscopy refers to the use of an image intensifier (II) coupled to a video camera that converts the image from the output screen of the II into a video signal (analog data). This signal is sent to a television monitor where images are displayed at frame rates of at least 30 frames per second (fps) to provide the effect of motion [9, 11–14].

Digital fluoroscopy modes

There are two modes of DF:

1. Use of an II coupled to a digital imaging chain (II-based DF).
2. Use of digital FPDs.

II-based systems are being replaced by the FPD systems. These systems are capable of producing dynamic images that can be displayed and viewed in real time. For this reason, these detectors are sometimes referred to as *dynamic FPDs*.

II-Based digital fluoroscopy characteristics

A typical II-Based DF imaging chain is shown in Figure 6.8. The major technical components include the x-ray tube and generator, an II tube, the optical image distributor, a video camera, an ADC, a digital computer, a digital-to-analog converter (DAC), and finally, the television monitor. Each of these will be described briefly as follows:

1. The *x-ray tube* is a high-capacity tube which is pulsed in operation. The x-ray *generator* is a high-frequency generator and can provide high mA values that is 100 times higher than conventional fluoroscopy which uses low mA values (1–3 mA) [1]. The generator operation is such that provides a pulsed x-ray beam, and this is often referred to as "pulsed-progressive fluoroscopy" [1]. Another important point that is noteworthy in DF is that "during digital fluoroscopy, the x-ray tube operates in the radiographic mode" [1].
2. The *video camera* used in II-based DF can be either a television camera tube or a charge-coupled device (CCD). If television camera tubes are used, they must have a higher SNR such as 1000 : 1 compared to 100 : 1 for tubes used in conventional fluoroscopy, and they

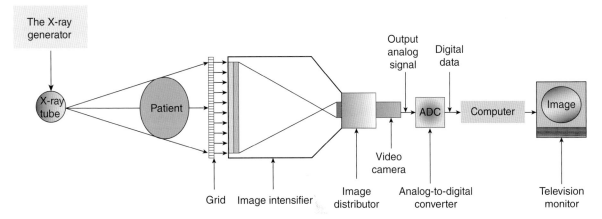

Figure 6.8 The major technical components of a typical II-based DF imaging chain include the x-ray tube and generator, an image intensifier tube, the optical image distributor, a video camera, an analog-to-digital converter (ADC), a digital computer, a digital-to-analog converter (DAC), and finally, the television monitor.

must also have low image lag. The CCD camera is now used in DF systems using IIs. The CCD has extremely high sensitivity and low readout noise level. CCDs can acquire images at 60/s compared with 30/s for television tubes.

3. The II tube provides *image intensification* which is defined as the brightening of the fluoroscopic image compared to the brightness obtained from a conventional fluorescent screen of the early fluoroscopes.

- The components of the II tube and their layout are shown in Figure 6.9. These include the input screen, photocathode, electrostatic lens, and an output screen, all enclosed in an evacuated glass envelope.
- The input screen is coated with a phosphor that converts x-ray photons to light photons. The state-of-the-art phosphor is CsI. The CsI phosphor absorbs twice as much radiation compared with ZnCdS, and is packed in a needle-like fashion (structured phosphor) to reduce the lateral spread of light in an effort to improve the spatial resolution compared with powdered CsI phosphors. The diameter of the input screen is variable; however, diameters ranging from 13 to 30 cm are not uncommon. Larger diameter IIs (36–57 cm) have become available for imaging larger anatomical regions such as the abdomen for example.
- The light emitted from the input screen strikes the photocathode which is made of cesium (Cs) and antimony (Sb) compounds and which emits photoelectrons. Multialkali photocathodes with a combination of potassium, sodium, and cesium will emit about three times more photoelectrons than Sb and Cs photocathodes, making these IIs much more efficient that single alkali photocathodes.
- The electrostatic lens or electron optics, as it is often referred to, consists of a series of electrodes that accelerate and focus the photoelectrons from the photocathode to the output screen. This requires a voltage of about 25–30 kV applied between the photocathode and the output screen.
- The output screen is coated with ZnCdS phosphor that converts the photoelectrons into light. The diameter of the output screen is about one-tenth the diameter of the input screen. Due to the acceleration of the photoelectrons and the small size of the output

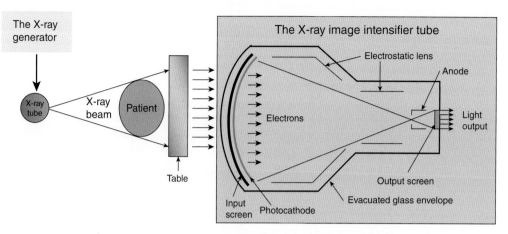

Figure 6.9   The components of the II tube and their layout include the input screen, photocathode, electrostatic lens, and an output screen, all enclosed in an evacuated glass envelope.

screen, the image at the output screen is extremely bright. This increase in brightness is conveniently referred to as brightness gain (BG).

$$BG = \text{minification gain}(MG) \times \text{flux gain}(FG).$$

- The glass envelope of the II tube is enclosed in a metal housing which not only provides mechanical support for the glass envelope, but also shields the intensifier against magnetic fields. Since the housing is lined with lead, it also shields from any radiation scattered within the glass envelope.
- The purpose of the image distributor is to split the total light (100%) from the output screen using a system of lenses and a beam splitting mirror, 10% of the light goes to the video camera, and 90% of the light goes to the photospot film camera, if such camera is used.
- *Magnification* of the image in conventional fluoroscopy is an important feature of the II. The purpose of magnification fluoroscopy is to enhance the image in order to facilitate diagnostic interpretation.
- Magnification fluoroscopy is only possible with multi-field IIs. These include the popular dual-field and the triple-field intensifiers that use a technique referred to as electron optical magnification [1]. This technique changes the voltage on specific electrodes of the electrostatic lens system in the II tube, to cause the electron beam crossover point to increase its distance from the output screen. A dual-field intensifier (25 cm/17 cm) can operate in the full-field mode (25 cm) and in the magnification mode (17 cm). When the magnification mode is used, the x-ray beam is automatically collimated to fall upon the central portion of the input screen to cover a diameter of 17 cm. On the other hand, a triple-field intensifier (25 cm/17 cm/12 cm) can operate in two magnification modes, 17 and 12 cm modes. The 12 cm mode provides greater magnification than the 17 cm mode.
- Magnification improves spatial resolution but at the expense of increased dose to the patient. Furthermore, the increase is about 2.2 times that used in the full-field mode of operation.

4. The *ADC* receives the output video signal (analog signal) from the video camera. This signal must be converted into digital data for processing by the computer. The process of digitizing the analog signal requires dividing it (the signal) into a number of parts. The unit of the parts is the bit (Chapter 2). A bit can be a 1 or it can be a 0. A 2-bit ADC will divide a signal into 4 (2^2) parts. Similarly, a 10-bit ADC will divide the signal into 1024 (2^{10}) parts. The higher the number of bits, the more accurate is the ADC.

5. A *digital host computer* is used in all DF systems. It is a minicomputer system capable of receiving dynamic digital data from the ADC and processing it quickly for image display. Data are received from the ADC in a matrix format generally with matrix sizes of 512×512 and 1024×1024. Each pixel in the image contains the atomic number and mass density characteristic of the tissue and represented by a single number for the pixel. The matrix is transformed into a gray scale image which can be described by the "bit depth" which refers to the number of shades of gray that a single pixel in the matrix (image) can assume. For example, while in a 3-bit depth image, each pixel can have 8 (2^3) shades of gray; an 8-bit depth image will provide 256 (2^8) shades of gray for each pixel, and so on. It is interesting to note that the spatial resolution of a digital image depends on the pixel size. As the pixel size decreases, the image appears sharper as the matrix size increases for the same field-of-view (FOV).

Flat-panel digital fluoroscopy characteristics

II-Based DF systems pose limitations related to artifacts. Such artifacts include image lag (continued emission of light from the screen when the radiation beam has been turned off), vignetting (loss of brightness at the periphery of the image, while the image is sharper and much brighter in the central portion of the screen), and veiling glare (scattering of light in the intensifier tube). Furthermore, there are other artifacts such as pincushion distortion (due to the curvature of the input screen in the II tube) and the 'S' distortion (Figure 6.10a) appears if an electromagnetic field is close to the intensifier (such as from a magnetic resonance imaging system). These distortions are eliminated by a flat-panel DF (FPDF) system, as illustrated in Figure 6.10b. The fundamental characteristics of a FPDF system will be described further.

The *major system components* of a FPDF imaging system (real-time imaging) are shown in Figure 6.11. The major difference between this system and the II-Based DF system (Figure 6.8) is the presence of the FPD. FPDs used in radiographic imaging produce static images and are therefore referred to as static FPDs. One significant and important technical characteristic of an FPD for fluoroscopy is that it must be capable of producing dynamic images that can be displayed and viewed in real time. For this reason, these detectors are sometimes referred to as *dynamic FPDs*.

The components shown in Figure 6.11 include the x-ray tube, patient, grid, the dynamic FPD, the host computer, and the television display monitor. The next section of this chapter will only highlight the basics of the *dynamic FPD*. There are two types of dynamic FPDs available for DF, namely, the *cesium iodide amorphous-silicon (CsI a-Si) TFT indirect digital detector* and the *a-Selenium TFT direct digital detector*. A major consideration of these detectors is that of a high frame rate and data transfer rate. Frame rates of 15–30 fps or greater are possible at readout speeds of 30–50 ms. Furthermore, dynamic FPDs can operate in at least two readout modes, namely, fps in continuous x-ray mode and fps in the pulsed x-ray mode. The overall goal of the latter is to reduce the dose to the patient during the examination.

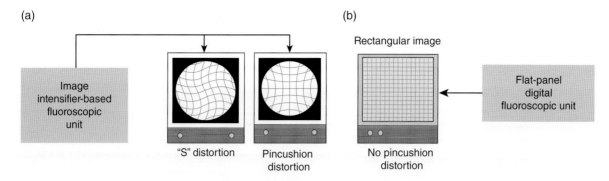

Figure 6.10 Artifacts such as pincushion distortion (due to the curvature of the input screen in the II tube) and the 'S' distortion (a) appears if an electromagnetic field is close to the intensifier (such as from a magnetic resonance imaging system). These distortions are eliminated by a flat-panel DF (FPDF) system, as illustrated in (b).

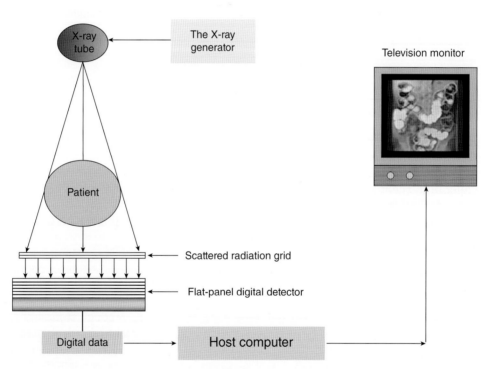

Figure 6.11 The major system components of a FPDF imaging system (real-time imaging). See text for further details.

A *dynamic FPD* must perform three elements in at least 33 ms for accurate performance in fluoroscopy. These include initialization, integration, and readout [15]. While initialization prepares the detector electronics for x-ray exposure, integration and readout are intended to collect the detector signal (analog signal) for subsequent digitization and image display. Another characteristic feature of these detectors is that of image magnification. In this regard, there are two methods used: (i) *electronic magnification* (zoom) and (ii) *binning*. With the former approach, there is no increase in spatial resolution and both original and magnified images have the same

SNR ratio. Binning has the disadvantage of less spatial resolution because the effective area of each image pixel is four times larger, and it has the advantage of lower data rates and less image mottle than ungrouped pixels.

FPD DF offers several advantages such as images free of distortion, improved contrast resolution, high DQE, uniform image quality over the whole displayed rectangular image, as illustrated in Figure 6.10b.

DF makes use of several image postprocessing operations such as gray scale image manipulation, temporal frame averaging, last image hold (lih), and edge enhancement. While gray scale image manipulation changes the contrast and brightness of an image displayed on the monitor, lih is intended to display the last frame continuously when the x-ray beam is turned off as a dose reduction strategy. Temporal frame averaging is a technique to reduce the image noise "by continuously displaying an image that is created by averaging the current frame with one or more previous frames of digital fluoroscopic image data" [16]. For example, averaging five frames will reduce the noise by about 44%; however, as more and more frames are averaged, image lag results. Finally, edge enhancement is an image sharpening technique [3].

DIGITAL MAMMOGRAPHY

Mammography is defined as radiography of the breast, and it is a prime example of soft tissue radiography, since the breast is composed of soft tissues such as adipose (fat), fibrous, and glandular tissues. To image the breast, the x-ray system must be capable of producing an x-ray beam that allows for maximum x-ray absorption by the soft tissues, microcalcifications, and thin fibers so that they can be shown on an image that shows excellent spatial resolution or detail.

Furthermore, mammography must be able to show the contrast between a lesion that is located in the breast and the normal anatomy that is around that lesion.

Mammography has evolved from screen-film mammography (SFM) and full-field digital mammography (FFDM) to DBT. The basics of each of these will be described further.

Screen-film mammography – basic principles

The major components of a *screen-film mammography* imaging system include a dedicated x-ray tube and generator, a special film-screen cassette designed to create optimum images of soft tissues of the breast, a chemical processor (wet chemistry), and a light view-box to display the film image for viewing and interpretation by a radiologist. When imaging, the radiation passes through the patient's breast to create a latent image on the film. The film is processed using chemical solutions to render the latent image visible.

Imaging system characteristics
It is not within the scope of this book to describe details of the mammographic imaging system, and therefore the interested reader must refer to other good radiography science books [9, 11] for a more complete account of important technical features. The imaging system features [1]:

- A high-frequency generator operating at 5–10 kiloHertz (kHz) with a voltage ripple of about 1%, with a maximum limit of 600 mAs in order to control patient dose.
- The x-ray tube is specially designed to produce low energy x-rays (soft x-rays) needed to image the soft tissues of the breast. For example, target/filter combination includes Tungsten/60 μm Molybdenum (Mo), Mo/30 μm Mo, Mo/50 μm Rhodium (Rh), and Rh/50 μm Rh. The x-ray

emission spectrum for Mo and Rh targets with relevant coupling of filter materials produce the appropriate spectrum. For example, "Bremsstrahlung x-rays are produced more easily in target atoms with high Z than in target atoms of low Z. Molybdenum and Rhodium K-characteristic x-rays have energy corresponding to their respective K-shell electron binding energy. This is within the range of energy that is most effective for breast imaging" [1]. Typical dimensions of the large and small focal spot sizes of the x-ray tube are 0.3 and 0.1 mm, respectively.

- The tube is operated at about low kV between 20 and 35 kV in 1 kV increments being commonplace.
- Typical grid ratios and grid frequency are 3 : 1 to 5 : 1, and 30 lines/cm.
- Automatic exposure control is used in order to deal with tissue thickness and composition as well as reciprocity law failure [1].
- The source-to-image receptor distance typically range from 50 to 80 cm.
- Breast compression is an essential procedural operation. The overall goal of such compression is to improve spatial and contrast resolution while reducing the dose to the breast tissues. It is important to note that "the breast tissue most sensitive to cancer induction by radiation is glandular tissue" [1]. The spatial resolution is about 15–20 line pairs/mm (lp/mm) limiting resolution which is needed to detect specks of calcium hydroxyapatite (microcalcifications) with diameters of around 0.01 mm (100 μm) [1].

Limitations of SFM

Despite the advantages of SFM, there are several shortcomings of SFM such as:

- Limited dynamic range of film due to its narrow exposure latitude. Film will only respond to a narrow range of exposures, and therefore the technologist must be extremely careful in selection of the optimum exposure factors to provide the best image contrast.
- The display characteristics of film such as its brightness and contrast are fixed once the film is developed in the chemical processor. Should the radiologist require other film images that are lighter or darker, then the technologist must perform the exam again using different exposure techniques.
- Another limitation of SFM is that the film serves three roles: acquisition, display, and storage.

Full-field digital mammography – major elements

DM solves the problems of FSM. FFDM is radiograph of the breast using a digital detector coupled to a digital computer that makes use of digital image processing techniques to enhance the visibility of detail and contrast of the image, in an effort to improve the detectability of breast lesions [17]. As reported by previous authors [17, 18], the advantages of FFDM summarized by Seeram [3] are as follows: wider dynamic range (while SFM offers a dynamic range of about 40 : 1, it is 1000 : 1 for FFDM); greater contrast resolution especially for dense breast tissue; use of digital image postprocessing operations to enhance image quality; the ability to communicate with a picture archiving and communication system (PACS); computer-aided detection (CAD) and diagnosis; DBT; and contrast-enhanced DM.

Imaging system characteristics

DM involves at least five fundamental steps: data acquisition, ADC, digital image processing, image display, image storage, archiving, and communications via the PACS. Data acquisition involves the use of digital detectors to collect the transmitted beam from the patient, convert the attenuation into digital data for processing by the computer. The following are noteworthy points to consider when reviewing FFDM system components:

- Three commonplace types of digital detector systems are used for FFDM, and these include the flat-panel phosphor system (cesium iodide amorphous silicon [CsI/a-Si]); flat-panel a-Se system, and a CR FFDM system (see Chapters 2 and 6). These detector systems must be capable of high spatial resolution needed for mammography imaging. Recall that FSM offers a spatial resolution of about 20 lp/mm. FFDM detectors must be capable of at least 10 lp/mm to improve lesion detectability [1] and must have an image area of at least 24 × 30 cm in order to capture the entire breast. Since the pixel size affects the spatial resolution, pixels must be spaced about 25 μm (0.025 mm) apart. Detectors must also have high SNR and a high DQE [17, 18].
- Applications of FFDM which are intended to assist in not only the detection of breast cancer but also to enhance the diagnostic interpretation skills of the radiologist. These include CAD and diagnosis, DBT, and contrast-enhanced DM. While CAD involves the use of the computer as a tool to provide additional information to the radiologist in order to make a diagnosis, and acts as a "second opinion," DBT is a three-dimensional (3D) mammography technique which uses special tomographic technique to overcome tissue superposition. Contrast-enhanced DM can be used in angiogenesis (appearance of new vasculature in a tumor) by using iodinated contrast medium.

DIGITAL TOMOSYNTHESIS AT A GLANCE

The fundamental problem with conventional mammography which produces two-dimensional (2D) images (produced by superimposed structures) is that it is difficult to clearly visualize specific pathologies of interest to the observer. The solution to this problem is digital tomosynthesis (DT), a 3D imaging technique that separates out the superimposed tissues. A more complete definition is that DT "is a three-dimensional imaging technique based on the reconstruction of several planar radiographs. During the image acquisition in tomosynthesis, the x-ray tube moves around the detector which is often stationary, and a number of projection images are taken from different angles. Individual slices from the reconstructed volume can be studied. With the effective reduction of the visibility of the overlapping normal tissue, the detection of pathological lesions is improved when compared with projection radiography" [19].

DT techniques have been applied in several clinical areas including orthopedics, angiography, chest, and breast imaging. In radiographic applications (chest, skeletal, head, and neck, emergency, and abdominal radiography), the technique can be referred to as radiographic tomosynthesis. Specifically, DBT has received increasing attention in the literature. DBT is "an extension of digital mammography that produces quasi three-dimensional reconstructed images from a set of low-dose X-ray projections acquired over a limited angular range."

Imaging system characteristics

The fundamental process of DT includes at least three steps, namely, data acquisition, image reconstruction, and image display on a workstation as illustrated in Figure 6.12.

- Data acquisition involves movement of the x-ray tube through various angles (θ = sweep angles), while the digital detector remains stationary (Figure 6.13).
- Image reconstruction algorithms (filtered back projection or iterative reconstruction algorithms) and digital image processing are used not only create DT images but also to enhance the visualization of image features, respectively.

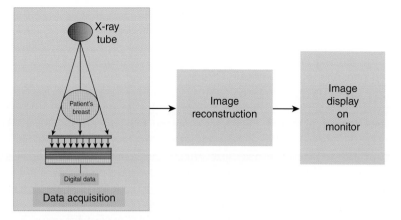

Figure 6.12 The fundamental process of digital tomosynthesis includes at least three steps, namely, data acquisition, image reconstruction, and image display on a workstation.

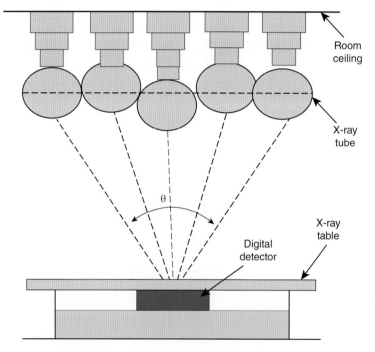

Figure 6.13 The fundamental principles of DT. See text for further explanation. *Source:* Yew and Seeram [20]. Licensed under CC BY 4.0.

- Image display monitors for DM must be calibrated and approved by the Food and Drug Administration (FDA) and must be calibrated, and have at least 5 million pixels, and meet luminance standards of the American College of Radiology (ACR).
- DT has found clinical applications in the chest, head, neck, and breast imaging (DBT) as well as in orthopedic, emergency, and abdominal imaging [20]. The reader should refer to Seeram [3] and Tingberg [19] for a more detailed description of DBT imaging principles.
- DT is also characterized by several parameters, which technologists must know. These include the sweep angle, sweep direction, patient barrier–object distance, number of

projections, and total radiation dose. The definitions of each of these as provided by Machida et al. [21] are as follows:

○ Sweep angle: *"This refers to the total arc about the center of the detector as defined by the focal spot position from the first to the final projection in the tomosynthesis acquisition or sweep. A sweep angle of 40° signifies a −20° to +20° sweep. The sweep angle can be varied between 20° and 40° on our flat-panel detector system."*

○ Sweep direction: *"The direction of X-ray tube movement relative to the object or body part of interest during a sweep. Sweep direction can be arbitrarily determined by altering the position or direction of the object or body part."*

○ Patient barrier–object distance: *"Is the minimum distance between the surface of the patient barrier and the object of interest. Detector–object distance should be used for more accurate geometric analysis, but patient barrier–object distance is convenient because it can be determined more easily and accurately."*

○ Number of projections and projection density: *"The number of projections is simply the number of X-ray projection images acquired during a single sweep. The projections are acquired at approximately constant angle intervals. For example, with a 40° sweep with 40 projections, a projection is acquired every 1°. As mentioned earlier, any number of projections from 25 to 60 can be selected on our flat-panel detector system. Projection density (number of projections divided by sweep angle) is used as an important conceptual parameter in the minimization of ripple artifact."*

○ Total radiation dose: *"Is the cumulative sum of the doses for all projections."*

Synthesized 2D digital mammography

An important technical advance in DBT is the production of a synthetic 2D image which can be generated from the DBT data set. This operation is referred to as *synthesized 2D digital mammography*. The process for generating a synthesized 2D image from the DBT image data is shown in Figure 6.14. First, DBT data acquisition is performed followed by the reconstruction of DBT 3D images. Next, the DBT 3D images are stacked and subsequently subjected to a synthesized 2D algorithm to generate synthesized 2D images. For additional details of synthesized 2D DM, the interested reader should refer to the work of Smith [22].

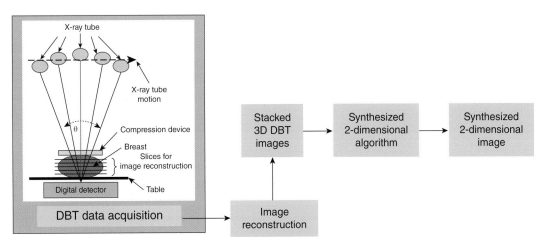

Figure 6.14   The process for generating a synthesized 2D image from the DBT image data. See text for further explanation.

References

1. Rowlands, J.A. (2002). The physics of computed radiography. *Physics in Medicine and Biology* 47: R123–R166.
2. Neitzel, U. (2005). Status and prospects of digital detector technology for CR and DR. *Radiation Dosimetry* 14 (1–3): 32–38.
3. Seeram, E. (2019). *Digital Radiography: Physical Principles and Quality Control*. Singapore: Springer.
4. Fuji Photo Film Company (2002). *Fuji Computed Radiography Technical Review. No 14, Imaging Plate (IP)*. Tokyo, 1–23
5. Seibert, J.A. (2004). Computed radiography technology 2004. In: *Specifications, Performance, and Quality Assurance of Radiographic and Fluoroscopic Systems in the Digital Era* (eds. L.W. Goldman and M.V. Yester). College Park, MD: American Association of Physicists in Medicine (AAPM).
6. Seibert, J.A. and Morin, R.L. (2011). The standardized exposure index for digital radiography: an opportunity for optimization of radiation dose to the pediatric population. *Pediatric Radiology* 41: 573–581.
7. International Electrotechnical Commission (2008). *IEC 62494-1 Ed. 1 Medical Electrical Equipment Exposure Index of Digital X-Ray Imaging Systems Part 1: Definitions and Requirements for General Radiography*. Geneva: IEC.
8. American Association of Physicists in Medicine (AAPM) (2009). An Exposure Indicator for Digital Radiography. College Park, MD: AAPM. *Report No. 116*.
9. Bushong, S. (2017). *Radiologic Science for Technologists*, 11e. St Louis: Elsevier-Mosby.
10. Willis, C.E., Thompson, S.K., and Shepard, S.J. (2004). Artifacts and misadventures in digital radiography. *Applied Radiology* 33 (1): 11–20.
11. Bushberg, J.T., Seibert, J.A., Leidholdt, E.M. Jr., and Boone, J.M. (2012). *The Essential Physics of Medical Imaging*, 3e. Philadelphia: Lippincott Williams and Wilkins.
12. Nickoloff, E.L. (2011). Survey of modern fluoroscopy imaging: flat-panel detectors versus image intensifiers and more. *Radiographics* 31: 591–602.
13. Seeram, E. and Brennan, P. (2017). *Radiation Protection in Diagnostic X-Ray Imaging*. Burlington, MA: James & Bartlett Learning.
14. Jones, A.K., Balter, S., Rauch, P., and Wagner, L.K. (2014). Medical imaging using ionizing radiation: optimization of dose and image quality in fluoroscopy. *Medical Physics* 41 (1): 014301. https://doi.org/10.1118/1.4835495.
15. Holmes, D.R., Laskey, W.K. et al. (2004). Flat-panel detectors in the cardiac catheterization laboratory: revolution or evolution—what are the issues? *Catheterization and Cardiovascular Interventions* 63: 324–330.
16. Pooley, R.A., McKinney, M.I., and Miller, D.A. (2001). Digital fluoroscopy. *Radiographics* 21: 521–534.
17. Mahesh, M. (2004). Digital mammography-physics tutorial for residents. *Radiographics* 24: 1747–1760.
18. Pisano, E. (2000). Current status of full-field digital mammography. *Radiology* 214: 26–28.
19. Tingberg, A. (2010). X-Ray tomosynthesis: a review of its use for breast and chest imaging. *Radiologic Clinics of North America* 52: 489–497.
20. Yew, S. and Seeram, E. (2020). Digital tomosynthesis: applications in general radiography. *Radiology Open Journal* 4 (1): 23–29.
21. Machida, H., Yuhara, T., Mori, T. et al. (2010). Whole-body clinical applications of digital tomosynthesis. *Radiographics* 30: 549–562.
22. Smith A (2016). Synthesized 2D mammographic imaging. White paper. Hologic, Inc™, Bedford, MA.

7

Image quality and dose

Diagnostic medical images contain information about the anatomical and functional details of a patient that can be used for making a diagnosis of the any medical condition of that patient. There are several metrics that go into producing that are used to describe *image quality* that allow the observer to conclude that the images are of diagnostic quality. These metrics apply to different imaging systems, such as film-screen radiography (FSR), computed radiography (CR), flat-panel digital radiography (FPDR), and computed tomography (CT), and are characterized by contrast resolution, spatial resolution, noise, detective quantum efficiency (DQE), and artifacts. Furthermore, while image quality is a central consideration in interpreting images, equally important is the radiation dose required to produce images of diagnostic quality; it is known that radiation exposure may or may not lead to biological effects. Radiation dose and biological effects will be outlined in Chapter 11. This chapter will focus on image quality metrics.

A Comprehensive Guide to Radiographic Sciences and Technology, First Edition. Euclid Seeram.
© 2021 John Wiley & Sons Ltd. Published 2021 by John Wiley & Sons Ltd.

THE PROCESS OF CREATING AN IMAGE

Figure 7.1 illustrates the process of creating an image of diagnostic quality. Achieving this goal requires several important elements. First, the imaging system (FSR, CR, FPDR, or CT) must be capable of transferring the structures in the patient onto the image. Second, this function depends on the physics of the imaging system to perform this task. As can be seen, the imaging system transfers two major classes of information: dose and image quality. The image quality characteristics transferred are contrast, sharpness, or detail, the amount of x-ray photons used to create the image. These characteristics are defined by the metrics of contrast resolution, spatial resolution, and noise, respectively. Additionally, the image detector plays a significant role in the transfer process based on its efficiency in converting the input dose to a useful image. This function is characterized by the metric referred to as the DQE. Finally, the imaging system will transfer any "any false visual feature on a medical image that simulates tissue or obscures tissue" [1] or equivalently "a feature in an image that masks or mimics a clinical feature" [2]. These are referred to as artifacts which can be disturbing to radiologists and may even result in an inaccurate diagnosis.

Third, with respect to Figure 7.1, the operator interacts with the imaging system to establish the correct technical factors to enable the transfer of the anatomy and other details onto the image to create a diagnostic image. Two of these factors, for example, are the dose to the patient which is partly determined by the exposure technique, mAs and kV (Figure 7.2), and the sensitivity of the image detector. In determining these factors, the operator must work within the International Commission on Radiological Protection (ICRP) as low as reasonably achievable (ALARA) philosophy, which simply means that the dose must be low as possible so as not to compromise the quality of the image.

Apart from the exposure technique, and the sensitivity of the image detector (or image receptor), there are other factors affecting the dose to the patient. For example, these include filtration, collimation and field size, scattered radiation grids, and the source-to-image receptor distance (SID), and will be described in Chapter 11.

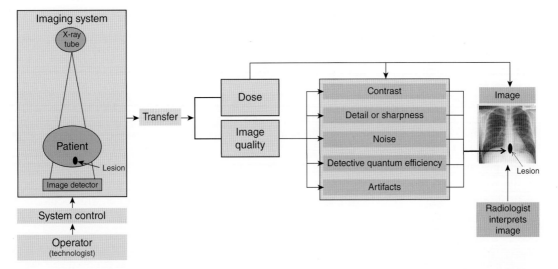

Figure 7.1   The process of creating a diagnostic quality image. The goal of the imaging system components is to transfer the lesion in the patient to the image displayed for viewing and interpretation without compromising the image quality.

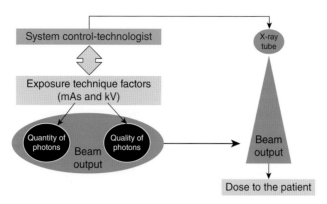

Figure 7.2 Technical exposure factors such as mAs and kV affect the dose to the patient to enable the transfer of the anatomy and other details onto the image to create a diagnostic image. Another factor is the sensitivity of the image detector.

IMAGE QUALITY METRICS

Contrast

Contrast falls into two categories, namely, *subject contrast* and *image contrast*, as illustrated in Figure 7.3. Since the image is displayed on a monitor for viewing and interpretation, sometimes it is referred to as *displayed contrast*. As noted by Wolbarst et al. [3], "contrast refers to the degree to which physical differences among materials within a body are revealed in the image. That is, contrast is an indication of the extent to which an organ, particularly tissue, or other object stands out from the background of other, nearby, and perhaps overlapping structures." In x-ray imaging (FSR, CR, FPDR, CT, and Fluoroscopy), contrast is created from the following sources: differential attenuation of the photons that occurs in the tissues due to their thickness, density, chemical composition (atomic number, Z), and the physics of the interaction of photons with tissues; that is, photoelectric absorption and Compton scattering (photon energy = kV). Figure 7.3 therefore illustrates the difference between subject contrast (arising from the difference in the density, Z) and image contrast (arising from the interaction of x-ray with matter, namely, based on the kV used, the value of which determines photoelectric effect [low kV] or the Compton effect [high kV]). These effects were described in Chapter 3.

Subject contrast is defined as "the difference in the x-ray intensities transmitted through a lesion and the adjacent structures" [4]. *Image contrast* on the other hand is defined as "the difference in intensity of a lesion in the image, in comparison to the intensity of the adjacent tissues. Image contrast is the result of subject contrast, together with the effect of the recording device and the image display characteristics" [4]. With respect to contrast, the following points are noteworthy:

- Contrast is improved with increasing object thickness, and the greater the difference in densities of objects.
- At lower kV techniques, the photoelectric effect predominates and therefore contrast is greater than at high kV techniques.
- At higher kV techniques, Compton effect predominates and therefore contrast is reduced at lower kV techniques.
- Contrast is improved if structures with higher Z values are imaged.

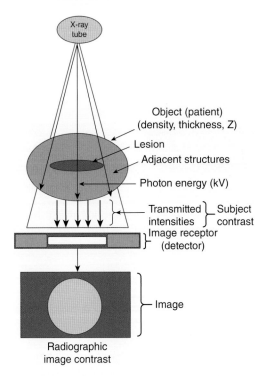

Figure 7.3   A schematic illustrating the difference between subject contrast (arising from the difference in the density, Z) and image contrast (arising from the interaction of x-ray with matter, namely, based on the kV used, the value of which determines photoelectric effect [low kV] or the Compton effect [high kV]).

- Increased scattered radiation will degrade contrast.
- Contrast can be improved with the use of anti-scatter grids. A high ratio grid is more efficient at removing scatter than low ratio grids and therefore improves contrast. High ratio grids, however, result in increasing dose to the patient.
- With digital radiography modalities and CT, image contrast can be changed by the operator using digital image postprocessing, most notably, the technique of windowing (Chapter 5). Figure 7.4 illustrates how the windowing can be used to alter the contrast of the image. Windowing will be described in more detail in Chapter 9.

Contrast resolution

The above description of contrast now leads to a definition of the term *contrast resolution*. Several authors have stated what is meant by contrast resolution. For example, Bushong [5] notes that contrast resolution is "the ability to distinguish anatomical structures of similar subject contrast such as liver–spleen and gray matter–white matter. The actual size of objects that can be imaged is always smaller under conditions of high subject contrast, than under conditions of low subject contrast." Another example is provided by Bushberg et al. [6], who states that contrast resolution "refers to the ability to detect very subtle changes in gray scale and distinguish them from the noise in the image. . .is not a concept that is focussed on physically small objects per se (that is the concept of spatial resolution); rather, contrast resolution relates more to anatomical structures that produce small changes in signal intensity (image gray scale) which makes it difficult for the radiologist to pick out (detect) that

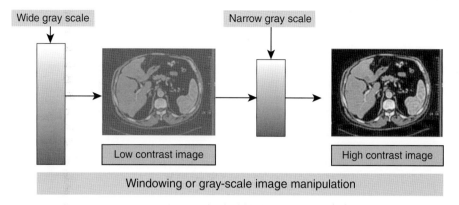

Figure 7.4 In digital radiography, contrast resolution is described by the gray scale of the image referred to as the dynamic range and it is the number of shades of gray that the imaging system can demonstrate. Windowing is a digital image processing operation that is used to change the image gray scale.

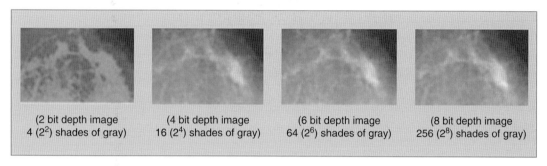

Figure 7.5 The effect of bit depth on the visual appearance of shades of gray of the image. As the bit depth increases, visual appearance improves.

structure from a noisy background." Yet another example is provided by Morin and Mahesh [7] who state that contrast resolution is used "to determine how well the imaging system faithfully renders the actual contrast in the structure being imaged. This could be viewed as the signal in the measured signal-to-noise ratio." The signal-to-noise ratio (SNR) will be described later in this chapter.

In digital radiography, contrast resolution is described by the gray scale of the image (Figure 7.4) referred to as the *dynamic range* [5] and it is the number of shades of gray that the imaging system can demonstrate. This range of gray shades is sometimes referred to as the density resolution of a digital image, which is linked to the *bit depth*; that is, the number of gray levels that a pixel can assume. An image with a bit depth of 8 would have 256 (2^8) shades of gray per pixel. Furthermore, a bit depth image of 10 would mean that each pixel can assume 1024 (2^{10}) shades of gray. The effect of bit depth on the visual appearance of shades of gray of the image is shown in Figure 7.5. As the bit depth increases, visual appearance improves.

Since the human eye can only perceive about 30 shades of gray [5], digital image post-processing would allow the human observer to see all shades of gray (256, 1024, and so forth). It is important to note as well that digital radiography detectors have a wide dynamic range, the major advantage being that the detector can respond to different levels of exposure (low to high) and still provide an image that appears acceptable to the observer, after preprocessing to correct the raw digital data obtained from the detector; and postprocessing to optimize the display of the image (contrast and sharpness enhancement) while noise can be reduced.

Spatial resolution

The patient's anatomy consists of large structures (vertebral bodies) and small structures (tiny calcifications, trabecular patterns in bone) which are transferred to the image by the imaging system during the imaging process. Figure 7.6 shows two chest images. While Figure 7.6a shows a sharp image, Figure 7.6b shows a blurred image. It is clear that visibility of fine details is much better in Figure 7.6a, than in the blurred image.

Spatial resolution is the ability of the imaging system to resolve fine details present in the object (patient), and refers to the sharpness of the structures that are close together and seen as distinct items on the image [4, 5, 8, 9]. Spatial resolution can also refer to the degree of blurring of structures in the image, and does not depend on exposure technique factors such as the kV and mAs [8].

The major factors affecting spatial resolution in radiography are the size of the x-ray tube focal spot, the area and thickness of the x-ray image receptor (detector), and movement of the patient during the x-ray exposure. While a small focal spot will produce sharper images than a large focal spot [10], as illustrated in Figure 7.7 (image of a bar pattern), thicker detectors (absorbing layer) generally produce less-sharp images (image blurring) [10]. Receptor (detector) blur originates in a manner in which the phosphor used in the detector is deposited. Recall Chapter 4 which described the indirect FPDR. The phosphor is deposited in a turbid (powdered) and in a structured (needle-like) fashion. While the turbid phosphor design results in a lateral spread of light, the structured phosphor "needle-like" design reduces the lateral spread of light which serves to improve the spatial resolution of the image [11].

Movement of the patient causes image blur. In addition, the following points about spatial resolution are important:

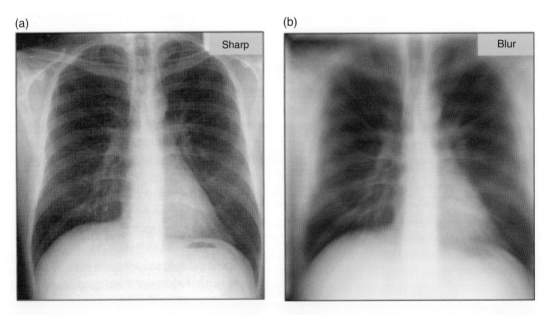

Figure 7.6 Illustration of spatial resolution. While (a) shows a sharp image, (b) shows a blurred image. It is clear that visibility of fine details is much better in (a), than in the blurred image.

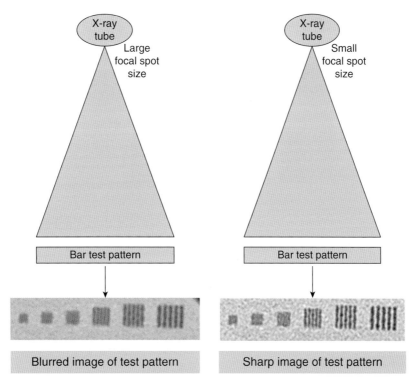

Figure 7.7 The size of the x-ray tube focal spot influences the spatial sharpness of an image. A small focal spot will produce sharper images compared to a large focal spot.

- Spatial resolution can be measured by metrics such as the *line pairs per millimeter* (lp/mm) and the more mathematically involved, *modulation transfer function* (MTF). A line pair consists of a black line (opaque) and a white line of equal size (Figure 7.8). Higher line pairs produce sharper images, hence better spatial resolution. For example, the spatial resolution (lp/mm) for mammography, radiography, CR, FPDR, fluoroscopy, and CT are 15, 8, 6, 4, 3, and 1.5, respectively [5]. The higher the lp/mm means that the closer the objects are to each other, and are smaller in size [8].
- The human eye can resolve about 5 lp/mm at a viewing distance of 25 cm [9].
- The limiting spatial resolution of an imaging system is the maximum number of lp/mm that the system is capable of demonstrating [5].
- Spatial resolution can also be described by the concept of *spatial frequency*. An image with a high lp/mm is a high spatial frequency image, since there are several alternating black and white regions/mm. In the patient, while fine structures produce high spatial frequencies (detail information), large objects will produce low spatial frequencies (contrast information). Another metric used to measure spatial resolution is the MTF of the system. The MTF is beyond the scope of this chapter; however, the following points are relevant and would aid the technologist in a better understanding of the performance of digital radiographic equipment.
  - Quality control (QC) bar test patterns with varying degrees of spatial frequencies (lp/mm) can be used to construct a modulation transfer function (MTF) curve by measuring the modulation (variation in strength) of each spatial frequency pattern, using a microdensitometer [5].
  - Plotting the modulation as a function of spatial frequency produces an MTF curve, and "10% MTF often is identified as the system spatial resolution" [5].

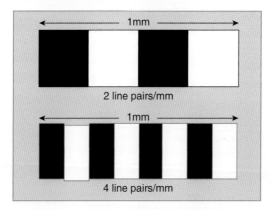

Figure 7.8 Spatial resolution can be measured by metrics such as the line pairs per millimeter (lp/mm). A line pair consists of a black line (opaque) and a white line of equal size. 4 lp/mm will produce a sharper image compared to 2 lp/mm.

- ○ The MTF curve can also show the limiting spatial resolution of the system.
- ○ Huda [4] notes that "at low spatial frequencies, the MTF is close to one, and corresponds to excellent visibility of relatively large features. At high spatial frequencies, the MTF falls to zero, which corresponds to the poor visibility of small features."
- An MTF of one represents a perfect transfer of spatial and contrast information [5].
- For digital imaging systems, the spatial resolution depends on the size of the pixels in the matrix. Smaller pixels will produce images with better spatial resolution compared with larger pixels. "Digital radiographs generally have a matrix size of 2000×2500. For a 35×43-cm cassette, this digital matrix corresponds to a pixel size of 175 μm and a limiting resolution of three line pairs per millimeter. For a 20×24-cm cassette, the pixel size would be 100 μm, and the limiting resolution would be five line pairs per millimeter" [9].

Noise

Figure 7.9 illustrates two images that show a change on the brightness across the images from, say, left to right in the absence of image detail. The change in the brightness is usually random and does not show any specific pattern; however, "in many cases it reduces image quality and is especially significant when the objects being imaged are small and have relatively low contrast. This random variation in image brightness is designated noise" [12]. Figure 7.9a and b shows two images with different levels of noise. Figure 7.9a shows an image with more noise compared to Figure 7.9b. It is clear that the image with more noise appears grainy, snowy, mottled, or textured. The image with less noise appears smooth and visually pleasing to look at. These characteristics are clearly demonstrated in Figure 7.9c and d which shows partial anatomical images of the chest. The presence of noise in an image destroys image quality and affects the visibility of low contrast objects, as illustrated in Figure 7.10a and b are two images of a 2×5 matrix imaged from a 10×10 matrix of circular indents (ranging from large to small) from a Contrast-Detail Quality Control Test Tool. While Figure 7.10b shows a noiseless image where all the circular indents are clearly visible, Figure 7.10a shows a noisy image in which the smaller circular indents cannot be clearly visualized. This phenomenon demonstrates that the visualization of low contrast objects (smaller circular indents) is limited by the presence of noise.

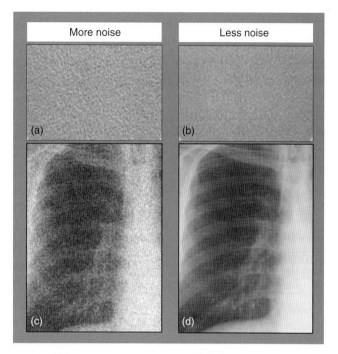

Figure 7.9 Two images with different levels of noise. (a) Shows an image with more noise compared to (b). It is clear that the image with more noise appears grainy, snowy, mottled, or textured. The image with less noise appears smooth and visually pleasing to look at. These characteristics are clearly demonstrated in (c, d) which shows partial anatomical images of the chest.

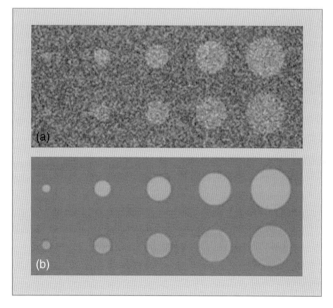

Figure 7.10 The presence of noise in an image destroys image quality and affects the visibility of low contrast objects. While (b) shows a noiseless image where all the circular indents are clearly visible, (a) shows a noisy image in which the smaller circular indents cannot be clearly visualized.

The concept of quantum noise

There are several sources of noise in radiographic imaging and these include electronic noise (due to the electronics of the system), detector noise (due to the physical characteristics of the detector), and quantum noise. Only the latter will be reviewed in this chapter.

The concept of quantum noise is illustrated in Figure 7.11. The photons from the x-ray tube fall upon the detector (image receptor) and are distributed in a random pattern. Such distribution results in what has always been referred to as *quantum noise*. The term quantum stems from the fact that each photon in the beam is a quantum of energy [5]. Quantum noise is determined by the number of photons (often referred to as the signal, S) used to produce the image. In Figure 7.11, two situations are illustrated, one in which there are 100 photons average per area (average of 100 photons per small square) and the other in which there are 1000 photons average per area (average of 1000 photons per small square). With this in mind, Sprawls [12] explains that "for a typical diagnostic x-ray beam, this is equivalent to receptor exposures of approximately 3.6 μR and 36 μR respectively." Furthermore, the number of photons per area in Figure 7.11a ranges from low (89) to high (114) and in Figure 7.11b, the range is from low (964) to high (1046). This variation of the values can be best expressed using the standard deviation (SD) which describes the amount of variation in the numbers. The SD is obtained by taking the square root of the average concentration of photons per area. Therefore, while the SD in Figure 7.11a is 10, the SD in Figure 7.11b is 33.3. The latter has a larger numerical value, than the former, and shows that there is a higher photon fluctuation (more noise). If this situation is expressed as a percentage, however, it computes to 3.3%, and demonstrates that the latter situation has less noise. "More specifically, quantum noise is inversely proportional to the square root of the exposure to the receptor" [12].

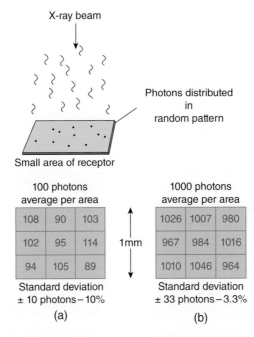

Figure 7.11 The concept of quantum noise. The photons from the x-ray tube fall upon the detector (image receptor) and are distributed in a random pattern. Such distribution results in what has always been referred to as quantum noise. *Source*: Courtesy of Dr. Perry Sprawls, PhD Professor Emeritus. Emory University.

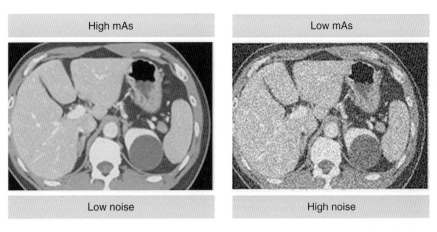

Figure 7.12   The visual effect of high and low mAs on image noise. See text for further explanation.

Low exposure technique factors (kV and mAs) will produce few photons at the receptor detector (less signal, S, and more noise, N); higher exposure technique factors will generate more photons at the detector (more S and less N). The former will result in a noisy image (grainy image) that is generally a poor image, and the latter will produce a better image at the expense of increased dose to the patient. The noise increases as the detector exposure decreases. The relationship between noise and mAs for the most part is that noise is inversely proportional to the square root of the mAs. Thus, if the mAs is reduced by a factor of 2, the noise increases by a factor of the square root of 2 (1.414 or 41%) [12]. Figure 7.12 illustrates the visual effect of high and low mAs on image noise.

Contrast-to noise ratio

In order to visualize a lesion, it is important that there is enough contrast (C) in the image compared to the amount of noise (N) present. If the noise can be reduced, then visibility of lesions would be improved. The contrast-to-noise ratio (CNR) is another metric to describe image quality. Therefore, if CNR can be improved, then detecting the lesion on an image is enhanced [4].

Signal-to-noise ratio

The SNR is yet another metric used to describe image quality in general. Figure 7.13 provides a conceptual approach to understanding SNR. Figure 7.13 can be thought of consisting of two components: the number of photons that create the image (Figure 7.13a), and which represent the signal (S) and Figure 7.13b which shows an image of the x-ray beam itself created by the random distribution of photons, noise (N). The SNR (S/N) image is shown in Figure 7.13c. SNR is equal to the square root of S. Increasing S (the number of photons to that create the image) will increase the SNR and improve the visibility of various tissues. The exposure technique factors (Figures 7.2 and 7.12), for example, can be used to increase the SNR (reduce the noise present in the image), by increasing the mAs (since mA determines the quantity of photons from the tube). The result of this action is an improvement in image quality. The problem with the use of higher mAs techniques, however, is that of increased patient dose. Technologists must always strive to work within the ALARA philosophy; that is, to keep the dose as low as possible without compromising image quality.

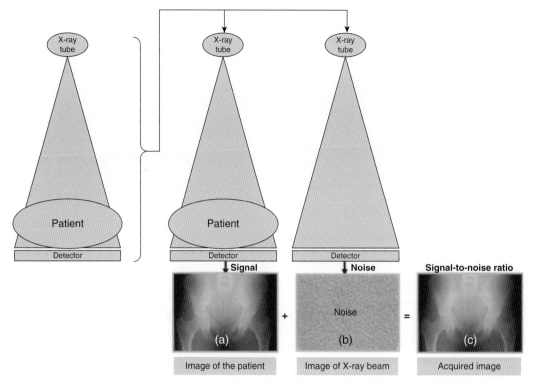

Figure 7.13   A conceptual approach to understanding SNR. See text for further details.

ARTIFACTS

Artifacts can degrade image quality and radiologists must be well-versed in identification of these artifacts since they can interfere with diagnostic interpretation. The definition of an artifact was given in Section "THE PROCESS OF CREATING AN IMAGE." A description of image artifacts is not within the scope of this chapter; however, the following points are noteworthy:

- Digital radiography is not free of artifacts.
- In general, CR artifacts arise from the image acquisition process and include operator errors and the image processing system as well [11, 13].
- The types of artifacts arising from the image acquisition and image processing systems as described by Shetty et al. [13].
- Flat-panel digital detectors are complex devices and pose numerous challenges in the manufacturing process. Flaws in the various components that make up the panel can lead to image artifacts.
- Several flaws, for example, include dust, scratches, chemical reactions of various materials that the detector is made of, and defective pixels.
- Image artifacts can also arise from vibrations or poor performance of the electronics and scattered radiation grids as well.

IMAGE QUALITY AND DOSE

Image quality and dose go hand in hand, since the dose is used to produce the desired image quality. Using the lowest possible dose without compromising the quality of the image is a basic tenet of the ALARA, one of the fundamental principles of radiation protection outlined by the ICRP.

Digital detector response to the dose

Figure 7.1 shows that the dose and image quality are linked, in that the dose affects several image quality parameters, such as contrast, noise, and DQE. Two important considerations in observing the ALARA principle are the response of the digital detector to the exposure, and how the detector deals with the noise. "Because of the statistical nature and distribution of radiation events, the noise is inversely related to the concentration of photons or exposure reaching the receptor. This relationship is crucial to arriving at the optimum exposure that provides the appropriate balance between image noise and patient dose" [10]. This is illustrated in Figure 7.14 for a digital radiography detector. Furthermore, the contrast-detail phantom images demonstrate visually that a high dose results in a higher SNR (less noise = better image quality) compared with the low dose image which results in an image with low SNR (more noise).

Since the detector response to dose is linear (Chapter 6), and because of image preprocessing inherent in the digital radiography imaging system, the dose does not affect image contrast, hence all three images appear visually the same. It is important, however, to recognize that while low doses produce images with high noise, higher doses produce images with less noise, and of course, better image quality. Therefore, a balance between image quality and dose is a challenging task for the

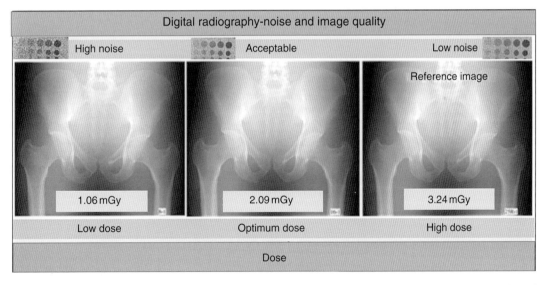

Figure 7.14 The relationship between image noise and patient dose, and visual image quality, for a digital radiography detector. Furthermore, the contrast-detail phantom images demonstrate visually that a high dose results in a higher SNR (less noise = better image quality) compared with the low dose image which results in an image with low SNR (more noise). The optimum goal in working within the ALARA philosophy is to obtain the optimum exposure that provides the lowest dose without compromising the image quality.

technologist using digital imaging equipment. The ultimate goal is to obtain an acceptable image with optimum dose (Figure 7.14) in order to operate successfully within the ALARA philosophy.

Detective quantum efficiency

The *DQE* is another useful metric in describing the performance of digital detectors in digital radiography. The DQE is a concept which deals with how efficient the detector is at converting radiation incident upon it (incident quanta) into a useful image signal that creates the image as shown in Figure 7.15. The DQE can be obtained using other physical quantities (MTF, noise power spectrum, the incident photon flux, photon energy, and spatial frequency). These quantities are beyond the scope of this textbook.

Figure 7.15 also shows that the DQE provides information about the SNR, and the goal is to demonstrate acceptable contrast resolution, in which case the signal is high and the noise is low. The following are noteworthy about the DQE:

- The DQE can be thought of as the efficiency of the digital detector to absorb, utilize, and preserve the x-ray image information.
- The DQE can be expressed as follows:

$$DQE = \frac{SNR_{out}^2}{SNR_{in}^2}.$$

- A perfect digital detector would have a DQE of 1.
- In general, the higher the DQE for a detector, the lower the image noise for a set amount of exposure, or equivalently.
- The higher the DQE for a detector, the lower the radiation exposure needed to achieve a set amount of image noise.
- The DQE values for indirect conversion cesium iodide (CsI) a-Si TFT flat-panel detectors offer the highest DQE at low frequencies. As the spatial frequencies increase, the DQE decreases rapidly [1].
- The DQE also depends on the photon energy (kV). Under controlled conditions it has been shown that the quantum efficiencies (based on the x-ray absorption properties of the detector converter materials) at 70 kV is about 67% for a-Se and 77% for CsI phosphor. At 120 kV, efficiencies are 37% for a-Se and 52% for CsI. In lower kV applications such as mammography, a-Se performs better than CsI and has a higher DQE [14].

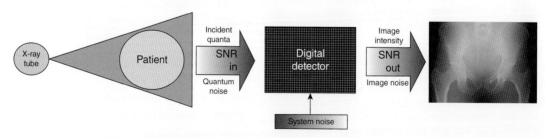

Figure 7.15   The DQE can be thought of as the efficiency of the digital detector to absorb, utilize, and preserve the x-ray image information. The DQE provides information about the SNR, and the goal is to demonstrate acceptable contrast resolution, in which case the signal is high and the noise is low.

References

1. Seibert, J.A. (2006). Computed radiography/digital radiography: adult. In: *RSNA Categorical Course in Diagnostic Radiology Physics: From Invisible to Visible-the Science and Practice of X-Ray Imaging and Radiation Dose Optimization* (eds. D.P. Frush and W. Huda), 57–71. Radiological Society of North America: Chicago, IL.

2. Willis, C.E., Thompson, S.K., and Shepard, S.J. (2004). Artifacts and misadventures in digital radiography. *Appl. Radiol.* 33 (1): 11–20.

3. Wolbarst, A.B., Capasso, P., and Wyant, A. (2013). *Medical Imaging-Essentials for Physicians*. Hoboken, NJ: Wiley.

4. Huda, W. (2016). *Review of Radiologic Physics*, 4e. Philadelphia: Wolters Kluwer.

5. Bushong, S. (2017). *Radiologic Science for Technologists*, 11e. St Louis, MO: Elsevier.

6. Bushberg, J.T., Seibert, J.A., Leidholdt, E.M. Jr., and Boone, J.M. (2012). *The Essential Physics of Medical Imaging*. Philadelphia, PA: Wolters Kluwer.

7. Morin, R.L. and Mahesh, M. (2018). Contrast resolution role in medical imaging. *JACR* 15 (7): 1002–1003.

8. Morin, R.L. and Mahesh, M. (2018). The importance of spatial resolution to medical imaging. *JACR* 15 (8): 1127.

9. Huda, W. and Abrahams, R.B. (2015). Ray-based medical imaging and resolution. *AJR* 204: W393–W397.

10. Sprawls, P. (2006). Radiographic image formation and characteristics. In: *RSNA Categorical Course in Diagnostic Radiology Physics: From Invisible to Visible. The Science and Practice of X-Ray Imaging and Radiation Dose Optimization* (eds. D. Frush and W. Huda), 9–28. Oak Brook, IL: Radiological Society of North America, Inc.

11. Seeram, E. (2019). *Digital Radiography-Physical Principles and Quality Control*. Springer Nature Singapore Pte Lid.

12. Sprawls, P. (1995). *Physical Principles of Medical Imaging*, 2e. Decatur, GA: Perry Sprawls and Associates Inc.

13. Shetty, C.M., Barthur, A., Kambadakone, A. et al. (2011). Computed radiography image artifacts revisited. *Am. J. Roentgenol.* 196: W37–W47.

14. Spahn, M. (2005). Flat detectors and their clinical applications. *Eur. Radiol.* 15: 1934–1147.

SECTION 3

Computed Tomography: Basic Physics and Technology

8

The essential technical aspects of computed tomography[1]

[1] Reprinted from Radiologic Technology, July/August 2014, Volume 85, Number 6. ©2014 by the American Society of Radiologic Technologists. All rights reserved. Used with permission of the ASRT for educational purposes. The original article title-Computed Tomography: A Technical Review.

Computed tomography (CT) is an extraordinary invention made possible through the work of several individuals, most notably Godfrey Newbold Hounsfield and Allan MacLeod Cormack. For their work, Hounsfield and Cormack shared the 1979 Nobel Prize in Medicine or Physiology [1]. The clinical benefits of CT evaluation and disease diagnosis are numerous and have continued to expand since the introduction of the technology in the early 1970s.

CT uses x-rays transmitted through the patient and to special detectors that convert the radiation beam into digital data for processing by a computer. The computer uses sophisticated algorithms called *image reconstruction techniques* to build up and display images of a patient's internal anatomy for diagnostic interpretation. These cross-sectional images are planar sections, or slices, that are perpendicular to the long axis of the patient. The technology used in CT has evolved from scanning a single slice to multiple slices in a single breath-hold. Current state-of-the art CT systems are based on volume data acquisition, in which the x-ray tube and detectors rotate continuously around the patient to gather transmission data from a volume of tissue rather than from one slice at a time. Volume-based technology expanded CT use to sophisticated applications in diagnostic CT imaging, along with nuclear medicine and radiation therapy.

CT scanners now can display a beating heart with excellent image quality and provide spectral information using dual-energy techniques. Furthermore, CT angiography, 3-D imaging, and virtual reality imaging are examples of clinical applications that have become commonplace in CT departments. Additionally, CT scanners are coupled with nuclear medicine equipment to create hybrid images, leading to molecular imaging which is "the visualization, characterization, and measurement of biological processes at the molecular and cellular levels in human and other living systems" [2]. Furthermore, CT imaging now forms the basis for radiation treatment planning or CT simulation.

The increasing use of CT has led to widespread concern about high patient radiation doses from CT examinations relative to other radiography examinations. Several efforts have focused on how to reduce patient dose and operate within the as low as reasonably achievable (ALARA) principle. Subsequently, a number of innovative tools have been developed by CT manufacturers, such as automatic exposure control (tube current modulation), automatic voltage selection (x-ray spectra optimization), more effective x-ray beam collimation, more efficient x-ray detectors, and more recently, image reconstruction techniques based on iterative reconstruction algorithms [3].

The purpose of this chapter is to outline the essential technical aspects of CT, ranging from the physics and technology of CT to image postprocessing, image quality, and radiation protection considerations.

BASIC PHYSICS

CT equipment acquires images using three primary system components (Figure 8.1). These include data acquisition, image reconstruction, and image display, storage, and communications. Data acquisition is the component in which the technology systematically scans a patient. Data acquisition involves an x-ray tube coupled to special electronic detectors. Image reconstruction creates images using sophisticated computer algorithms. Display, storage, and communication of processed images rely on digital technology. A microcomputer coupled with the display monitor supports interpreter manipulation using special image processing operations. Images are subsequently stored on magnetic or optical data carriers and can be communicated by electronic means to other locations. Finally, the images can be sent to remote locations using PACS (Picture Archiving and Communication Systems). An important element of data acquisition is that the x-ray tube and detectors rotate around the patient to systematically collect x-ray attenuation data that are then sent to the computer for reconstruction of CT images, as illustrated in Figure 8.2.

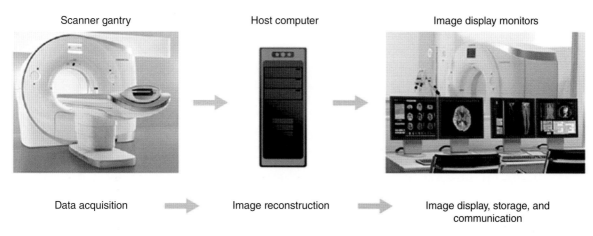

Figure 8.1 The computed tomography (CT) scanner consists of three primary system components for image production: data acquisition, image reconstruction, and image display, recording, storage, and communication systems. *Source*: Images courtesy of Siemens Healthcare GmbH and Euclid Seeram.

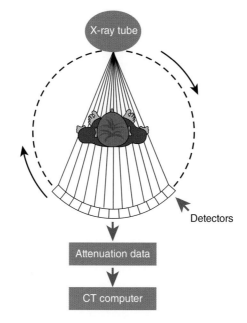

Figure 8.2 CT data collection. The x-ray tube and detectors rotate around the patient to systematically acquire x-ray attenuation data that are subsequently sent to the computer for image reconstruction. *Source*: Images reprinted with permission from the American Society of Radiologic Technologists. © ASRT 2020.

Radiation attenuation

Determining attenuation of the CT beam in a patient's tissues is complex and involves physics, mathematics, and computer science. Attenuation is the reduction of the radiation beam's intensity as it passes through an object. The object absorbs some photons, but other photons are scattered. Attenuation in CT depends on the effective atomic density (atoms/volume), the atomic number of the absorber, and the photon energy. There are two types of radiation beams: homogeneous and heterogeneous. In a homogeneous beam, all the photons have the same energy, yet the atoms have differing energies in a heterogeneous beam [1]. See Figure 8.3 for the attenuation behavior of each of these beams. Equal thicknesses of the object remove equal amounts of photons in a homogeneous beam, while the number of photons decreases (attenuation) through the object. The energy of the attenuated photons remains the same (see Figure 8.3a). The beam quantity changes, but the beam energy (quality) remains the same. The situation is different for a heterogeneous beam, in which equal thicknesses do not remove equal amounts of photons. This phenomenon results in a decrease in the number of photons (attenuation) through the object, but an increase in the energy of the attenuated photons (see Figure 8.3b). The heterogeneous beam's quantity and quality change [4]. Increasing the penetrating power of the photons hardens the beam. This effect is referred to as *beam hardening* and can create beam hardening artifacts on CT images. Beer–Lambert Law Attenuation of a homogeneous beam is exponential and can be described by the equation shown in Figure 8.4. During development of the CT scanner, Hounsfield used a gamma radiation source, not an x-ray tube. The gamma radiation emitted a homogeneous beam in his initial experiments because such a beam satisfies the requirements of the Beer–Lambert law [4–6]. This law is an exponential relationship described by the equation:

$$I = I_0 e^{-\mu x},$$

where I is the transmitted intensity; I_0 is the original intensity; e is Euler constant (2.718); μ is the linear attenuation coefficient, or the fractional reduction in the intensity of a beam of radiation per unit thickness of the medium traversed; and x is the thickness of the object. The fundamental problem in CT is to calculate the linear attenuation coefficient, expressed as μ, which indicates the amount of attenuation that has occurred. The equation $I = I_0 e^{-\mu x}$ can be solved to find the value of μ as follows [4–6]:

$$I = I_0 e^{-\mu x}$$
$$\ln I_0 / I = \mu x$$
$$\mu = (I / x) \cdot (\ln I_0 / I),$$

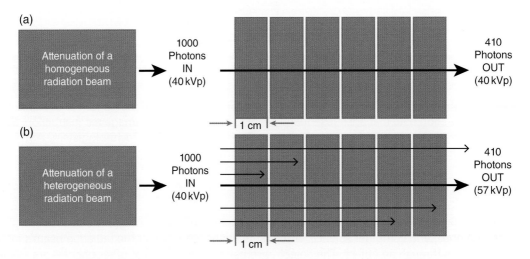

Figure 8.3   The difference between the attenuation behavior of two types of x-ray beams: a homogeneous beam (a) and a heterogeneous beam (b).

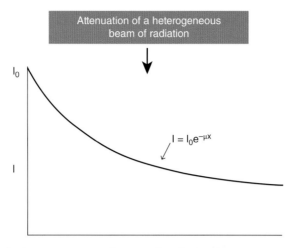

Attenuation of a heterogeneous
beam of radiation

$I = I_0 e^{-\mu x}$

Figure 8.4 Attenuation of a homogeneous beam of radiation is exponential and is described by the Beer–Lambert law.

where ln is the natural logarithm. In CT, however, the beam is attenuated by a given amount of tissue with a specific thickness Δx. Hence, the attenuation is expressed as:

$$I = I_0 e^{-\mu x}.$$

As the CT scanner's x-ray beam passes through a stack of volume elements, or voxels (see Figure 8.5), that is, part of the slice, the scanner obtains an attenuation measurement called a *ray sum* [4–6]. The ray sum is the total of all linear attenuation coefficients along the path of a single ray through the patient. In this situation, the transmitted intensity I is represented as [5]

$$I = I_0 e - \sum_{i=1}^{n} \mu_i \Delta X,$$

where

$$\sum_{i=1}^{n} \mu_i \Delta X = -\left(\mu_1 + \mu_2 + \mu_3 + \cdots \mu_n \right) \Delta X.$$

Taking the natural logarithm, this equation can be written as [5]

$$\ln\left(I_0 / I \right) = \sum_{i=1}^{n} \mu_i \Delta X.$$

Calculations of the linear attenuation coefficients in CT are challenging because the system must calculate each of the coefficients in the entire slice. The values of transmitted intensity and original intensity are known and are measured by detectors. Furthermore, change in thickness also is known so the system can calculate the linear attenuation coefficient. The image reconstruction process requires that the system obtains many ray sums for different locations (rotation angles) around the slice. A significant problem with the gamma source of radiation used by Hounsfield in his initial experiments was that the beam intensity was too low, and therefore, it took too long to scan and produce an image [1]. Hounsfield subsequently switched to a diagnostic x-ray tube. The beam from this tube is heterogeneous; the radiation's photons have a range of energies, which does not satisfy the Beer–Lambert law. As a result,

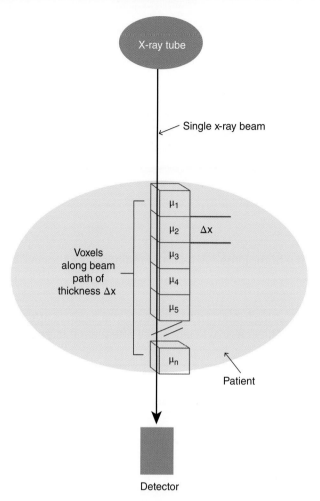

Figure 8.5 As a single ray of the x-ray beam passes through a stack of voxels, the CT system obtains an attenuation measurement called a ray sum. A ray sum is the sum of all μ's along the path of a single ray through the patient.

Hounsfield had to make several assumptions and adjustments to determine the linear attenuation coefficients. It is necessary to make the heterogeneous beam in CT approximate a homogeneous beam to satisfy the equation and solve for linear attenuation coefficient. Attenuation and CT Numbers: Each CT imaging slice consists of a matrix of voxels (e.g. 512×512 or 1024×1024). Figure 8.6 illustrates what happens to the attenuation through a single voxel. The attenuation value is converted into an integer (0, a positive number, a negative number) referred to as a *CT number* [1, 4–6]. The system subsequently normalizes all voxel values to the attenuation of water (μ_{water}). CT numbers are computed using the following algebraic expression [5, 6]:

$$CT\ number = \frac{\mu_{tissue} - \mu_{water}}{\mu_{water}} \cdot K,$$

where K is the scaling factor (contrast factor) of the CT manufacturer. In general, K is equal to 1000. The range of CT numbers produced using this factor is referred to as the Hounsfield (H)

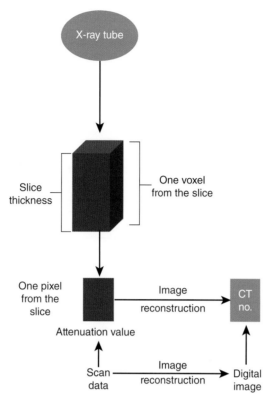

Figure 8.6   Attenuation through a single voxel. The attenuation value is converted into an integer (0, a positive or negative number) referred to as a CT number.

scale, which results in 0.1% per CT number [5, 6], thus expressing linear attenuation coefficients much more accurately compared with the scale used in pioneering CT units. CT numbers always are computed with reference to the attenuation of water. The CT number for water is 0, while it is 11 000 for bone and 21 000 for air on the Hounsfield scale. Linear attenuation coefficient values depend on several factors, including the beam energy [5, 6]. For example, μ_{water} at 60 keV is 0.206 cm^{-1}, but at 73 keV, 0.19 cm^{-1} is the linear attenuation coefficient [5, 6]. The original CT scanner used the latter value for water attenuation. See Table 8.1 for CT number ranges for bone, muscle, white matter, gray matter, blood, tumors, water, fat, lungs, and air. The CT equipment obtains a matrix of CT numbers for each image slice. These can be printed out as a numerical image. However, radiologists interpret from gray scale images, which require converting the numerical image into a gray-scale image as shown in Figure 8.7. CT numbers are referred to as *gray levels* [1] in digital image processing. Converting the numbers into shades of gray (*gray scale*) results in higher numbers assigned white, lower numbers black, and gray shades between black and white. This assignment is related to the attenuation characteristics of tissues. Bone attenuates more radiation and therefore is assigned white (the bone's appearance is the same on a film-screen image as it is on a digital image). Air attenuates very little radiation and appears black on film-screen and digital images. The range of CT numbers is defined as the *window width* (WW) and the center of the range is defined as the *window level* (WL). Finally, the radiologist can manipulate the WW to alter image contrast, and the WL to alter image brightness.

Table 8.1 Computed tomography number ranges.

Tissues	Range
Bone	800–3000
Muscle	35–50
Brain (white matter)	36–46
Brain (gray matter)	20–40
Blood	13–18
Tumors	5–35
Water	0
Fat	–100
Lungs	–150 to –400
Air	–1000

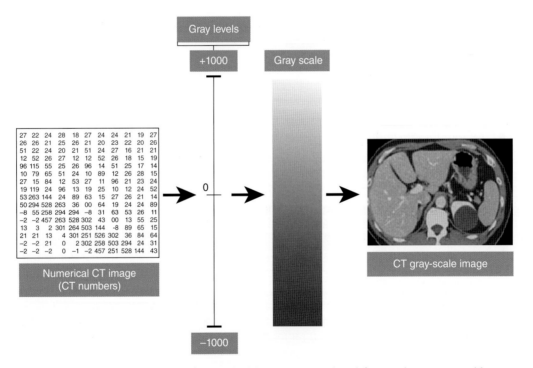

Figure 8.7 The matrix of CT numbers (numerical image = gray levels) must be converted into a gray-scale image for viewing by radiologists and technologists.

TECHNOLOGY

CT technology refers to the basic equipment configuration that consists of three primary systems (Figure 8.1): data acquisition, image reconstruction, and image display, storage, and communication systems.

Data acquisition: principles and components

Data acquisition is a systematic collection of attenuation data from the patient through various scanning methods. These methods have evolved from scanning one slice at a time during a single rotation of the x-ray tube and detectors to scanning multiple slices per single rotation of the x-ray tube and detectors (multislice CT [MSCT]) around the patient. MSCT scanners now are commonplace and rely on fan-beam geometry to scan the volume of tissue. The term *geometry,* or *data acquisition geometry,* refers to the size, shape, motion, and path traced by the x-ray beam [4]. The path is created by the patient moving through the gantry aperture during scanning and is called a *spiral* or *helical path.* MSCT scanners are based on spiral/helical beam geometry (Figure 8.8). The multislice scanners have evolved incrementally from 4 to 640 slices per revolution of the x-ray tube. The helical geometry improves the volume coverage speed without compro-

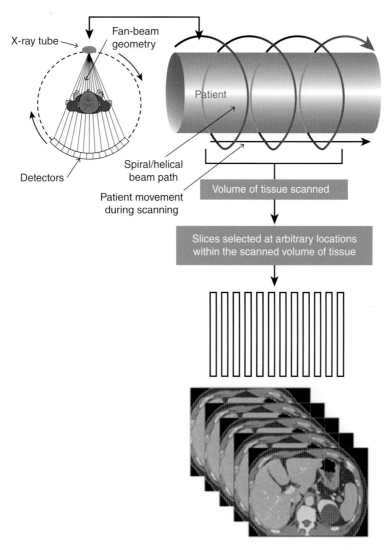

Figure 8.8 Multislice CT (MSCT) scanners use fan-beam geometry to scan the volume of tissue. *Source*: Images reprinted with permission from the American Society of Radiologic Technologists. © ASRT 2020. Euclid Seeram.

mising image quality. Several components housed in the scanner gantry acquire data (Figure 8.9). The x-ray tube and detectors rotate around the patient to collect multiple attenuation readings. The x-ray beam passes through a specially shaped filter called a *bow-tie filter* to make the beam more uniform at the detector and thus satisfy the Beer–Lambert law for calculating the linear attenuation coefficients. Collimation directs the beam through only the slice of interest and the detectors measure the transmitted photons, which subsequently are converted into digital data by the analog-to-digital converters. The digital data are sent to the computer for image reconstruction.

Image reconstruction

Image reconstruction is based on complex mathematics – the reason Godfrey Hounsfield shared his Nobel Prize with physicist and mathematician Allan Cormack. Images are reconstructed by producing a 2-D "distribution (usually of some physical property) from estimates of its line integrals along a finite number of lines of known locations" [7]. In CT, the physical property is the linear attenuation coefficient of the tissues, and the line integral refers to the sum of the attenuation along each ray in the beam that passes through the slice [7]. Image reconstruction uses algorithms, or defined rules for solving a problem, to systematically build an image during the scanning process. The algorithms used in CT include the earlier back-projection algorithm and newer analytic reconstruction techniques such as the filtered back-projection algorithm.

Filtered back projection
Basics consists of two main components: convolution filtering and subsequent back projection of the filtered profiles (Figure 8.10) [8, 9]. The early back-projection algorithm involves the summation of multiple back projections of data obtained with the x-ray source at various angles until reconstruction of the complete image. However, the final reconstructed image is blurred

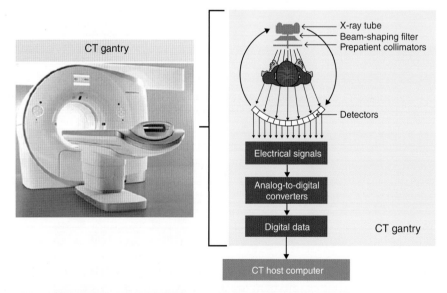

Figure 8.9 Primary components of a CT scanner data acquisition system: the x-ray tube, filter, collimator, patient, detectors, and detector electronics that include the analog-to-digital converter. *Source*: Images reprinted with permission from the American Society of Radiologic Technologists. © ASRT 2020. CT scanner Image courtesy 2017 Siemens Healthcare GmbH.

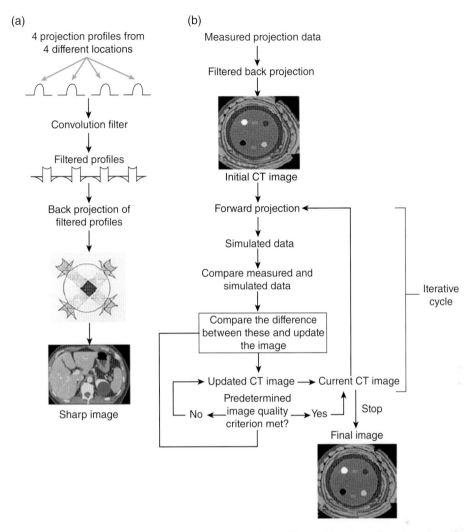

Figure 8.10 Flow charts showing the primary steps of the filtered back-projection algorithm (a) and a generic iterative reconstruction algorithm (b). Diagram courtesy of the author. CT images in (b). *Source*: (a) Euclid Seeram. (b). Image reprinted with permission from Kim et al. [53].

and useless. The filtered back-projection algorithm was developed to solve image blurring by applying convolution filtering (digital filter) to each set of projection data before back projection to improve sharpness and contrast [3, 8–12]. These convolution filters increase noise in images, especially in low-dose CT examinations, and are thus viewed as a limitation of the filtered back-projection algorithm. Other limitations of the filtered back-projection algorithm are based on underlying assumptions about scanner geometry, such as the use of pencil x-ray beam geometry, a point source x-ray focal spot (which is an approximation based on the assumption of its infinitely small size), failure to consider the shape and size of detector cells and voxels, and neglecting image noise resulting from Poisson statistical variations of x-ray photons [9, 12].

Iterative reconstruction

The introduction and widespread use of iterative reconstruction algorithms resulted from shortcomings of the filtered back-projection algorithm [3, 8–11]. With the development of

MSCT scanning, other algorithms were necessary to address the problems associated with the patient moving through the CT gantry during the scanning process as the x-ray tube and detectors rotate continuously around the patient. Iterative reconstruction algorithms, which first were used in the 1970s but were impractical for clinical use because of a lack of computational power, re-emerged and now are commonplace in CT scanners. These algorithms solve the problems of image artifacts and image noise generated by the filtered back-projection algorithm, especially in low-dose CT scanning [3]. Iterative reconstruction algorithms model the CT system more accurately, and subsequently improve image quality, especially for low-dose CT examinations. Iterative reconstruction algorithms therefore can reduce image noise while preserving image sharpness and contrast, especially at low tube currents. Iterative reconstruction algorithms also help reduce metal artifacts and beam hardening effects caused by photon starvation [9, 10, 12, 13]. CT manufacturers provide several different iterative reconstruction algorithms with their CT scanners. For example, GE Healthcare offers Adaptive Statistical Iterative Reconstruction (ASiR) and Model-Based Iterative Reconstruction (MBIR) [3]; Siemens Healthineers offers Iterative Reconstruction in Image Space (IRIS) and Sinogram Affirmed Iterative Reconstruction (SAFIRE). In addition, Philips offers iDose4, and Toshiba Medical Systems offers AIDR (Adaptive Iterative Dose Reduction), along with AIDR 3-D [3]. A generalized iterative reconstruction process is illustrated in Figure 8.10, including the following steps [3, 10, 12]:

1. During scanning, iterative reconstruction acquires measured projection data and then reconstructs the data using the standard filtered back-projection algorithm to produce an initial image estimate.
2. The initial image estimate then is forward projected to create simulated projection data (artificial raw data) that then are compared with the measured projection data.
3. The algorithm then determines differences between the two sets of data to generate an updated image that is back projected on the current CT image; this minimizes the difference between the current CT image and the measured projection data.
4. The user must evaluate image quality based on a predetermined criterion included in the algorithm.
5. If the image quality criterion is not met, the iteration process repeats several times in an iterative cycle until the difference is considered sufficiently minimal.
6. The final CT image matches quality criteria after the termination of the iterative cycle. A comparison of images reconstructed using filtered back projection and an iterative reconstruction algorithm is shown in Figure 8.11. Iterative reconstruction algorithms are common in modern-day MSCT scanners, especially for optimizing dose in children.

Image display, storage, and communication

The third main component of CT systems is the display of the reconstructed image for viewing and interpretation, along with postprocessing to suit the needs of the interpreting radiologist. Furthermore, images are sent to PACS for storage and communication to virtual data centers for retrospective analysis. Electronic communications in CT require a standard protocol that facilitates connectivity (networking) among imaging modalities and equipment from multiple manufacturers. The standard used for this purpose is DICOM (Digital Imaging and Communications in Medicine).

(a)

(b)

(c)

(d)

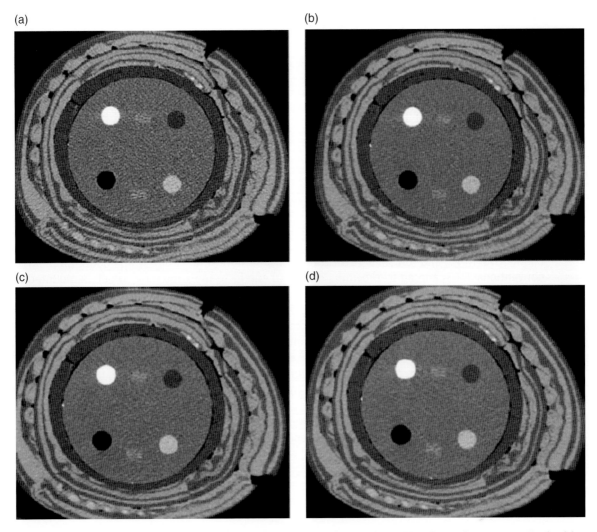

Figure 8.11 A visual comparison between CT images obtained at 180 mAs and reconstructed with filtered back projection (a) adaptive iterative dose reduction 3-D mild (b), 3-D standard (c), and 3-D strong modes (d). *Source*: Reprinted with permission from Kim [53].

MULTISLICE CT: PRINCIPLES AND TECHNOLOGY

MSCT evolved from single-slice CT, which overcame the limitations of conventional CT (stop-and-go, slice-by-slice data acquisition) by decreasing data acquisition time and thereby increasing the volume coverage speed. Other advantages of MSCT include isotropic spatial resolution, efficient use of the x-ray beam, reduced radiation exposure, and improved accuracy in needle placement for CT fluoroscopy and cardiac CT imaging. The strategy in MSCT is to acquire data continuously as the patient moves through the gantry and the x-ray tube and detectors rotate around the patient. This strategy requires special equipment considerations and several technical approaches such as [1, 4, 14]:

- Slip-ring technology and x-ray tubes that provide very high x-ray output.
- Interpolation algorithms.
- 2-D detector arrays.
- Continuous table movement.
- Mass computer memory buffer.

Slip-ring technology

Slip-ring technology enables scanning of a patient moving through the gantry, while the x-ray tube and detectors rotate continuously around the patient. Slip rings are electromechanical devices that transmit electrical energy across a rotating interface through circular electrical conductive rings and brushes [18]. Slip rings remove the cable wraparound problem of conventional CT scanning by providing electrical energy to the x-ray tube, which is mounted on the rotating frame of the gantry. The slip rings also transfer the signals from the detectors for input into the image reconstruction computer. The x-ray generator is mounted on the rotating frame and connects to the x-ray tube via a short piece of high-voltage cable. CT manufacturers offer two types of slip-ring scanners: low-voltage or high-voltage units. The two types differ in power supply to the slip ring. In the low-voltage system, the alternating current (AC) power and x-ray control signals are transmitted to slip rings through low-voltage brushes that glide in contact grooves on the stationary slip ring. The slip ring then provides power to the high-voltage transformer, which subsequently transmits high voltage to the x-ray tube [1]. In a high-voltage slip-ring system, the AC powers the high-voltage generator, which subsequently supplies high voltage to the slip ring. In this case, the generator does not rotate with the x-ray tube, and the x-ray generator, x-ray tube, and other controls are positioned on the orbital scan frame [1].

X-ray tube technology

A fundamental problem with conventional x-ray tubes is heat dissipation and slow cooling rates. Furthermore, as gantry rotation times increase, higher milliampere (mA) values are needed to provide the same mA per rotation. As the electrical load (mA and kilovolts, or kV) increases, the x-ray tube requires faster anode cooling rates. MSCT scanners require x-ray tubes that can sustain higher power levels because the tube rotates continuously for a longer period compared with conventional scanners. Several technical advances in component design have resolved these power levels and dealt with the problems of heat generation, storage, and dissipation. For example, the tube envelope, cathode assembly, anode assembly (including anode rotation), and target have been redesigned [15, 16]. X-ray tube issues have been addressed by the introduction of new tubes such as the Straton x-ray tube and more recently, the Vectron x-ray tube, both developed by Siemens Healthineers. These tubes are compact and use direct anode cooling technology, which results in high cooling rates and other technical advantages. Philips Healthcare has introduced the upgraded Maximus Rotalix Ceramic (iMRC) x-ray tube based on metal/ceramic technology. The iMRC also has a noiseless spiral-groove bearing with a large liquid metal contact and a 200-mm graphite-backed, dual suspended hydrodynamic bearing with a segmented all-metal anode disk to facilitate high heat-loading capacity and rapid heat dissipation.

Interpolation algorithms

In helical CT data acquisition, movement of the patient through the gantry aperture while the tube rotates around the patient can cause problems, including [1, 4, 6]:

- Difficulty localizing a specific slice because there is no defined slice as in conventional CT scanning (Figure 8.12).
- Slice volume geometry that is somewhat different than in conventional CT scanning (Figure 8.12).
- Increased effective slice thickness because of the width of the fan beam and the speed of the table.
- Inconsistent projection data because there is no defined slice. This is important because consistent data are needed to satisfy the filtered back-projection algorithm. If inconsistent data are used with this algorithm, the image displays streak artifacts similar to motion artifacts. Image reconstruction steps can overcome these problems. First, the system produces a planar section similar to the slice in conventional CT scanning. The planar section is generated using interpolation algorithms (Figure 8.12). Interpolation is a mathematical technique to estimate the value of a function from known values on either side of the function. Second, the images are reconstructed using the standard filtered back-projection algorithm. The results are CT images free of motion artifacts [1].

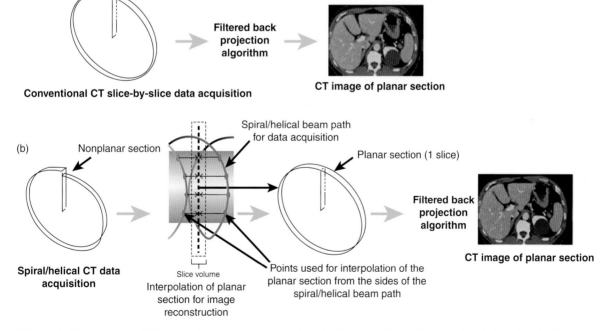

Figure 8.12 A main difference between conventional slice-by-slice CT scanning (a) and spiral/helical CT scanning (b) lies in the geometry of the slice.

MSCT detector technology

The detector is one of the most important components in the CT imaging chain because it captures radiation passing through the patient and converts it into electrical signals that subsequently are digitized and sent to the computer for processing and image building. Currently, two categories of detectors capture and convert radiation into digital data. These include scintillation detectors and photon-counting detectors.

The main components of the two types of scintillation detectors – the conventional energy integrating and dual-layer types – are shown in Figure 8.13. These are the most common detectors used in CT. The following are key points regarding CT detectors:

- Scintillation crystals convert x-ray photons to light photons, which then are converted to electrical signals by photodiodes. Detector electronics called *application-specific integrated circuits* (ASICs) digitize the signals [17].
- Scintillation crystals used in MSCT include cadmium tungstate (CdWO4); ceramic material made of high-purity, rare-earth oxides based on doped rare-earth compounds such as yttria; and gadolinium oxysulfide ultrafast ceramic. GE Healthcare has made use of gemstone spectral imaging. The GE Gemstone is the first garnet scintillator for use in CT. Furthermore, Philips Healthcare uses zinc selenide activated with tellurium in their dual-layer scintillator detectors [17].
- The photon-counting detector is an emerging technology that is being tested in prototype scanners such as the Siemens SOMATOM Definition Flash. These detectors use semiconductors such as cadmium telluride (CdTe) and cadmium zinc telluride (CZT) [18] because they can convert x-ray photons directly into electron hole pairs (electric charge) [19].

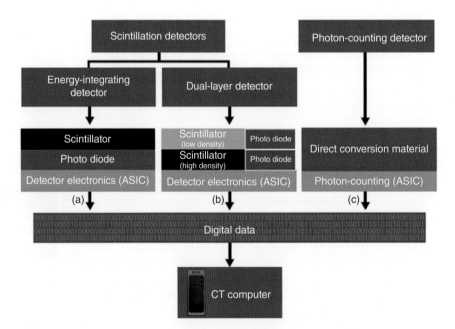

Figure 8.13　The main components of two types of scintillation detectors: conventional energy integrating detectors (a) and dual-layer detectors (b). The main components of the photon-counting detector or direct conversion are shown in (c). ASIC, application-specific integrated circuit.

One of the most important differences between single-slice CT and MSCT is the design of the detector. Single-slice detectors are based on a one-detector array design, and MSCT detectors are based on a 2-D design as illustrated in Figure 8.14. Whereas 1-D detector arrays acquire one slice per single rotation of the x-ray tube and detectors, 2-D detectors acquire several slices per single rotation of the x-ray tube and detectors during volume scanning. For example, a 2-D detector with 64 detector rows acquires 64 slices per single rotation. Two types of 2-D detector arrays are shown in Figure 8.15: matrix array and adaptive array. The detector designs are based on preferences of the CT manufacturer. The matrix array detector is divided into equal detector elements, and the adaptive array detector features pairs of equal elements. For example, the two central elements are equal, and the two elements closest to the central elements are equal to one another. Slice selection with 2-D detectors is based on the detector configuration used. According to Dalrymple et al., this configuration "describes the number of data collection channels and the effective section thickness determined by the data acquisition system settings" [20]. For example, in Figure 8.15a, each detector channel in the matrix array detector is 1.25 mm and four cells are activated or grouped (binned) together to produce four separate images of 1.25-mm thickness per 360° rotation.

Selectable scan parameters

The technologist can select several MSCT scanning parameters. These include the scan mode, exposure factors (kV, mA, and scan time), gantry rotation time, pitch, scan length, collimation, and slice width. In particular, pitch determines image quality needed and is related to patient dose. As pitch increases, the dose decreases but with degradation in image quality (Figure 8.16). Patient dose is inversely proportional to the pitch. The current universal definition of pitch for MSCT scanner technology is from the International Electrotechnical Commission [21]: the pitch (P) is equal to the

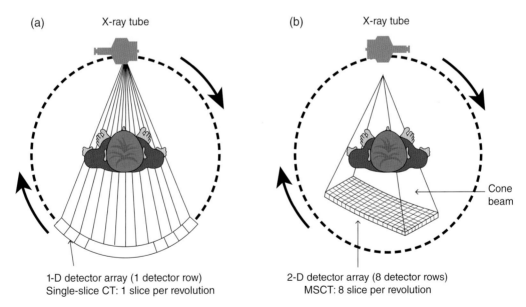

Figure 8.14 A main difference between single-slice CT and MSCT is the detector design. Single-slice detectors are based on a 1-D detector array design (a) and MSCT detectors are based on a 2-D design (b). *Source*: Images reprinted with permission from the American Society of Radiologic Technologists. © ASRT 2020.

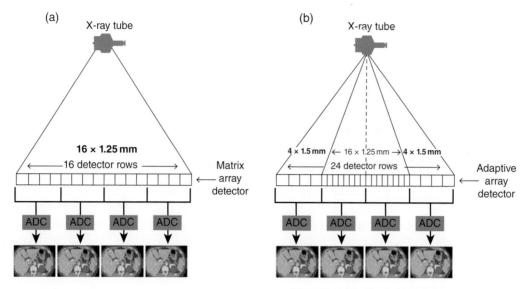

Figure 8.15 Two types of 2-D detector arrays used in MSCT scanners: the matrix array (a) and the adaptive array (b), and examples of binning the detector channels to obtain different slice thicknesses. ADC, analog-to-digital converter.

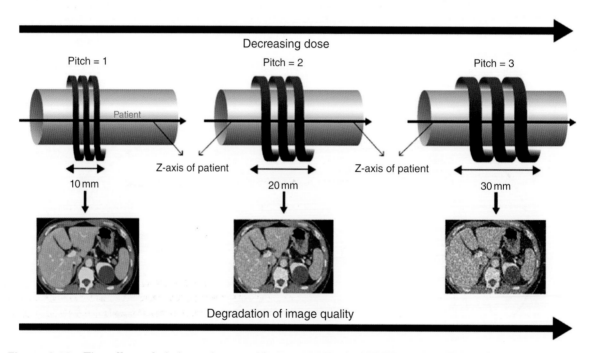

Figure 8.16 The effect of pitch on dose and image quality in MSCT. As the pitch increases, the dose decreases with a corresponding degradation of image quality. *Source*: Images reprinted with permission from the American Society of Radiologic Technologists. © ASRT 2020.

distance the table travels per rotation (d)/total collimation (W). The total collimation is equal to the number of slices (M) times the collimated slice thickness (S). Algebraically, the pitch is expressed as:

$$P = d / W \text{ or } P = d / M \times S.$$

Isotropic CT imaging

MSCT scanners have evolved from 4 to 640 slices per revolution of the x-ray tube and detectors around the patient. The purpose of this ongoing evolution coupled with other technical developments is to achieve isotropic spatial resolution, in which all dimensions of the voxel (*x, y, z*) are equal, and therefore the voxel is a perfect cube. Matrix array detectors are considered isotropic in design (cells equal in all dimensions). If all voxel dimensions are not equal, that is, the slice thickness is not equal to the pixel size, the data set acquired is anisotropic. Figure 8.17 shows the geometry of both isotropic and anisotropic voxels. The overall goal of isotropic imaging in CT is to achieve excellent spatial resolution in all imaging planes, especially when reconstructing multiplanar and 3-D images. Technologists should be aware that as the voxel size decreases, radiation dose increases [20].

MSCT image processing

Computer architectures for MSCT have evolved from an early pipeline processing system to the use of parallel and distributed processing architectures to accommodate more sophisticated processing and clinical application tasks. The specific architecture chosen for an MSCT system depends on how the computer assigns various tasks, such as preprocessing raw data; image reconstruction; display tasks, such as 3-D or virtual reality imaging; and purpose, such as CT angiography. Numerous processors in the computer's electronic circuits complete processing tasks. The MSCT computer rapidly processes the large data sets acquired and the high number of iterations needed to complete the computationally intensive reconstruction operations of CT iterative reconstruction algorithms. The need for rapid processing challenges the capacity of the central processing units of modern-day computers used in medical imaging and radiation therapy. Therefore, CT computer architecture also includes a graphics processing unit to reduce the processing requirements of the central processing unit. The graphics processing unit now contributes to image reconstruction, image processing, dose calculation and treatment plan

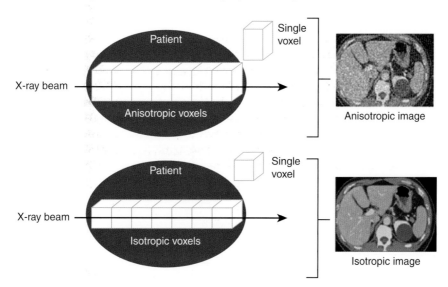

Figure 8.17 The geometry of isotropic and anisotropic voxels. The overall goal of isotropic imaging in CT is to achieve excellent spatial resolution in all imaging planes, especially when reconstructing multiplanar and 3-D images. *Source*: Seeram [1] © 2016, Elsevier.

optimization, radiation treatment planning, and other applications. Current graphics processing units can construct complex 3-D images in milliseconds [22].

IMAGE POSTPROCESSING

Three classes of software contribute to CT systems. These include image reconstruction, pre-processing, and image postprocessing software. Preprocessing software corrects data collected from the detectors before the data are sent to the reconstruction computer, and image post-processing software involves manipulating system is so sophisticated that it has been called *visualization and analysis software*, and consists of basic and advanced image display and analysis tools. Image postprocessing operations are called *image enhancement* [23, 24]. The purpose of image enhancement is to display an image according to some interpreter preferences and assist with diagnostic interpretation. Image enhancement operations include contrast and brightness enhancement, edge enhancement, spatial and frequency filtering, image combining, and noise reduction. The most popular of these operations for use in medical imaging is contrast and brightness enhancement, also called *windowing*.

Windowing

CT images are made up of a range of numbers (CT numbers). The range of numbers in the image is called the WW and the center of the range of numbers is called the WL. Digital image processing theory refers to the numbers as gray levels; these levels are converted into a gray scale to display the data as images rather than as numbers (Figure 8.7). WW controls image contrast, and WL controls the image brightness. A wider WW creates an image with less contrast, but a narrow WW provides improved image contrast (Figure 8.18). The effect of WL on image brightness is illustrated in Figure 8.19. As the WL increases and the WW remains constant

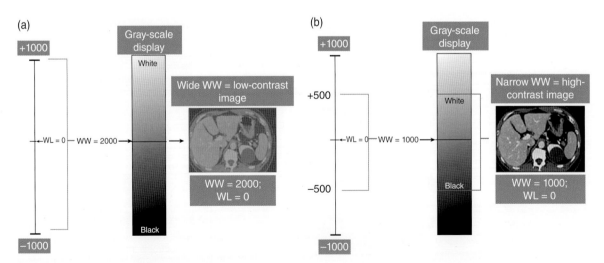

Figure 8.18 A graphic illustration of the effect of window width (WW) on a CT image. Window width controls image contrast, and window level controls image brightness. A wide window width shows an image with less contrast (a) and a narrow window width improves image contrast (b).

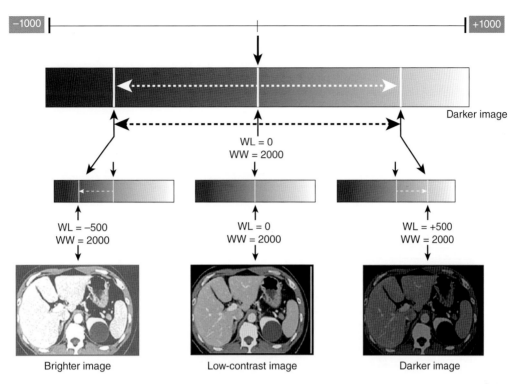

Figure 8.19 The effect of window level (WL) on image brightness. As the window level increases (keeping the window width constant [e.g. 1500]), the image becomes darker because more of the lower numbers are displayed. A lower WL (e.g. 2500) provides a brighter image because more of the higher CT numbers are displayed.

(e.g. to 1500), the image becomes darker because more of the lower numbers are displayed. A lower WL value (e.g. 2500) with WW remaining constant provides a brighter image because more of the higher CT numbers are displayed.

3-D image display techniques

The ability to display 3-D CT images has applications in evaluating the craniomaxillofacial complex; musculoskeletal system; central nervous system; and cardiovascular, pulmonary, gastrointestinal, and genitourinary systems. Display of CT scans in 3-D now is commonplace in CT angiography [25–29]. The use of 3-D visualization techniques is a type of digital image processing operation called *image synthesis*. The purpose of image synthesis is to create images that are useful when the desired image is impossible or impractical to acquire [30]. The 3-D display techniques are based on computer graphics principles and technology. At least four major elements are essential to creating 3-D images (Figure 8.20). The elements include CT image acquisition, creation of 3-D space, processing for 3-D image display, and 3-D image display for the interpreting physician or observer. The data collected from scanning the patient are used to create 3-D space, which contains all voxel information and is processed for 3-D image display. Processing 3-D CT images involves preprocessing, visualization, manipulation, and analysis. Surface- and volume-rendering techniques can transform 3-D space into simulated 3-D images for display on a 2-D computer monitor [25]. Surface rendering is a relatively simple operation in which the surface of an object is created using contour

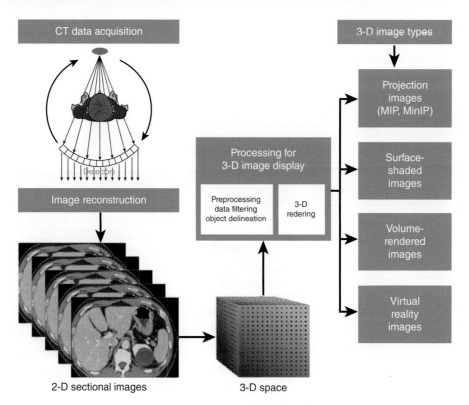

Figure 8.20　Creating 3-D CT images involves four primary steps: image acquisition, creation of 3-D space, processing for 3-D image display, and 3-D image display for the interpreting physician. MIP, maximum intensity projection; MinIP, minimum intensity projection. *Source*: Images reprinted with permission from the American Society of Radiologic Technologists. © ASRT 2020. Euclid Seeram.

data and shading of pixels to provide the illusion of depth. Surface rendering uses only 10% of the data in 3-D space and requires little computation. Volume rendering, on the other hand, is much more sophisticated; the technique uses all the data in 3-D space and requires more computational power. Maximum and minimum intensity projections, for example, are volume-rendering techniques that make use of only those voxels in 3-D space that have the maximum (brightness) or minimum values. These values are assigned to the pixels in the displayed maximum and minimum intensity projection images, which are used extensively in CT angiography.

IMAGE QUALITY

CT image quality, essential for diagnostic interpretation, is characterized by at least five physical parameters including spatial, contrast, and temporal resolution; noise; and artifacts [31, 32]. Spatial resolution is the fine detail or sharpness of objects seen in an image.

Spatial resolution

Spatial resolution also referred to as *high-contrast resolution*, is a CT scanner's ability to resolve closely spaced objects that are significantly different from their background, or to show small objects that have high subject contrast. Detail in digital images is influenced by the matrix size, field of view (FOV), and slice thickness. As a result, smaller pixel sizes provide images with greater detail for the same FOV. The pixel size can be calculated as follows:

$$\text{Pixel size}(p) = \text{FOV} / \text{matrix size}.$$

As slices become thinner, the degree of image sharpness increases. Radiography still demonstrates the best spatial resolution of all imaging modalities because the images can show object sizes of 0.1 mm compared with 0.5 mm for CT and magnetic resonance (MR) images, 2 mm for diagnostic medical sonograms, and 5 mm for nuclear medicine images [33].

Contrast resolution

Contrast resolution refers to the CT scanner's ability to display images with small differences in soft tissues expressed in millimeters at 0.5%. CT has much better contrast resolution than radiography, nuclear medicine, or sonography. However, MR imaging has superior contrast resolution to all imaging modalities. Contrast resolution for MR is 1 mm, compared with 20 mm for nuclear medicine, 10 mm for sonography, and 10 mm for radiography [33]. Imaging moving organs, such as a beating heart, has become routine; however, organ movement can cause imaging blurring. Temporal resolution describes the CT techniques used to detect movement over time and freeze the motion of organs. The techniques address the speed of data acquisition and are significant for cardiac CT and other applications that require reducing the effects of motion on images to achieve diagnostic quality [1].

Noise

Noise in CT is a random variation of CT numbers in the image of a water phantom. Several factors affect CT image noise, including the number of x-ray photons reaching the detectors, beam energy, voxel size, and slice thickness. For example, larger voxels in anisotropic imaging and thicker slices generate more noise than images with smaller voxels and thinner slices. A noisy image displays a grainy appearance (Figure 8.17) [1]. Artifacts are distortions or errors in an image that are unrelated to the object being imaged. Any discrepancy between the reconstructed CT image and the true attenuation coefficients of the object also is considered an artifact [34]. As noted by Barrett and Keat [34], the artifacts originate from one of several categories or causes: physics-based artifacts from the physical processes involved in CT data acquisition, patient-based artifacts from factors such as patient movement or metallic materials, scanner-based artifacts from scanner function imperfections, and helical and multisection artifacts, which are produced during image reconstruction.

RADIATION PROTECTION

Technological advances in CT scanner design and performance have contributed to increasing use of CT in clinical medicine. Numerous studies report higher patient doses from CT relative to other modalities [35–37]. For example, CT doses to each organ within the image field typically range from 5 to 50 mGy [38]. As of 2011, CT contributed the highest collective amount of medical radiation exposure in the United States compared with any other medical imaging modality [45]. High doses from pediatric CT examinations have called attention to the risks of cancer associated with CT scanning [45]. The literature stresses the need to optimize dose in CT.

The International Commission on Radiation Protection (ICRP) refers to optimization as keeping radiation doses ALARA to avoid compromising the diagnostic quality of an image. Optimization therefore addresses both radiation dose and image quality.

CT dosimetry

In CT, there are at least three dose metrics: the computed tomography dose index (CTDI), dose-length product (DLP), and effective dose. The CTDI and the DLP always appear on the dose report the CT console displays. Although CTDI and the DLP relate to patient dose, the effective dose relates the radiation exposure to risk and is considered the best method available to estimate stochastic radiation risk [39]. The CTDI is a standardized measure of radiation dose output of a CT scanner that helps the user to compare radiation output of various CT scanners. CTDI provides a measure of the exposure per slice of tissue and information about the amount of radiation used to perform the examination, which is reported in milligray (mGy). The use of a weighted CTDI ($CTDI_w$), the sum of the CTDI in the middle and periphery of the phantom that examines the average dose in the x–y axis of the patient, is computed as follows [1, 4–6]:

$$CTDI_{vol} = \frac{CTDI_w}{pitch}.$$

When the pitch is 1, the $CTDI_{vol}$ equals the $CTDI_w$. The $CTDI_{vol}$ is the same whether a technologist scans a 10- or 100-mm length of tissue, and therefore another metric is needed; this is the DLP. The DLP is a much more accurate representation of the dose for a defined length of tissue. The DLP measures the total dose for a CT scan (L equals the length of the scan in centimeters) along the patient's z axis and is expressed in mGy-cm. The DLP is directly proportional to the length of tissue scanned. The DLP is computed as follows:

$$DLP = CTDI_{vol} \times L.$$

Factors affecting patient dose

Several factors affect patient dose in CT; however, those that technologists can select to optimize dose are technique factors (mAs and kVp), pitch, collimation and slices, automatic exposure control, noise index, overbeaming (excess dose beyond the edge of detector rows per rotation of a multisection scan), over-ranging (use of additional rotations before and after the planned length of tissue so the first and last images can be reconstructed), and noise-reducing image reconstruction algorithms. In CT, the mAs per slice is called the *effective mAs* [40, 41]. In summary, patient dose is:

- Directly proportional to the square of the voltage (kV) change.
- Directly proportional to the mAs.
- Inversely proportional to the pitch.
- Increased as the collimation width (wider beam five thicker slices) increases.
- Increased with overbeaming and over-ranging.
- Related to the noise index; when the noise index is reduced by 5%, dose increases approximately 11%. If the noise index is increased by 5%, the dose is reduced by approximately 9% [41].
- Affected by the use of automatic tube current modulation. For example, Toth et al. [39] reported that the effective dose in chest CT examinations was reduced by approximately 10%. Further, longitudinal modulation accounts for two-thirds of dose reduction, and angular modulation accounts for the remaining one-third.

- Related to the use of iterative reconstruction algorithms. Several studies have demonstrated reductions in radiation dose from 30 to 50% using iterative reconstruction [41, 42]. Consensus is that iterative reconstruction algorithms can reduce radiation dose and improve image quality in CT compared with filtered back-projection algorithms [3].

Optimizing radiation protection

International and national radiation protection organizations and radiation safety campaigns have established regulatory and guidance documents and diagnostic reference-level recommendations. CT radiation protection regulatory and guidance recommendations are available from the ICRP, National Council on Radiation Protection and Measurements [43], U.S. Food and Drug Administration [44], and Health Canada [45]. Several campaigns also promote radiation awareness and safety worldwide. Two popular campaigns include Image Gently [46] and Image Wisely [47]. Another method of optimizing radiation protection in CT is the use of diagnostic reference levels. A diagnostic reference level is used as an investigational level to identify unusually high radiation doses for common diagnostic examinations [41]. The American College of Radiology, for example, recommends a diagnostic reference level for an adult CT abdomen and pelvis examination of 25–30 mGy and an adult chest CT of 21 mGy [41]. All professionals who work in CT should adhere to the optimization principles of the ICRP and work within ALARA principles. Radiologic technologists must play a significant role in reducing patient dose and protecting staff present during the examination. To be an effective participant in CT dose optimization, a radiologic technologist must have a thorough understanding of the elements listed in the Box 8.1 for optimizing dose.

Box 8.1
Essential elements for technologists to optimize CT dose

1. The risks of radiation and CT dose in particular.
2. Current technical advances in CT.
3. CT dose metrics, particularly $CTDI_{vol}$, the DLP and effective dose, and associated units.
4. CT image-quality metrics such as spatial resolution, contrast resolution, noise, and artifacts.
5. Technical factors affecting patient dose in CT including exposure technique factors, AEC, pitch, effective milliampere seconds, slice thickness, scan field-of-view, beam collimation, noise-reducing algorithms (iterative reconstruction algorithms), anatomical coverage, overbeaming, overranging, patient centering, and noise index.
6. Scan protocols and reviewing the protocols with the radiologist on an ongoing basis with the goal of optimizing dose and image quality.
7. The pre scan and postscan display of CT dose reports showing the $CTDI_{vol}$, DLP, and effective dose.
8. How to get involved with the development or implementation of a CT dose-monitoring or dose-tracking system for the CT department. Monitoring and tracking should include items such as dose capture, conversion of absorbed dose to effective dose, patient-specific storage, dose analytics, dose communication, and data export.
9. How to participate in research on CT patient dose and image quality optimization. This requires a fundamental knowledge of CT equipment and dosimeter calibration, image acquisition details, observer performance measures, and appropriate statistical tools.
10. How to ensure continuous professional development through relevant continuing education activities.

Abbreviations: AEC, automatic exposure control; CT, computed tomography; $CTDI_{vol}$, volume CT dose index; DLP, dose-length product.

Technologists also must continue to collaborate actively with radiologists and medical physicists to enhance competent and reflective operation of CT scanners [42].

CONCLUSION

As CT scans, and especially MSCT scans, increasingly support routine clinical diagnosis, advanced applications deserve attention. For example:

- Cardiac CT imaging, which has become commonplace in medical imaging departments. Imaging a beating heart with previous iterations of MSCT scanners resulted in image artifacts. In addition, organ coverage was limited by detector size (20–40 mm), which required at least two rotations to cover the entire organ and the lungs. These shortcomings are addressed by the 640-slice dynamic volume CT scanner and dual-source CT scanner [48, 49].
- The CT scanner now is used widely in radiation oncology and has become integral to the simulation process [50]. The CT simulation process includes several steps, such as scanning the patient in the CT scanner, planning the treatment and CT simulation, and setting up the patient in the treatment machine.
- Image fusion combines anatomical images from a CT scanner with functional images from nuclear medicine (positron emission tomography) or create a new synthesized image that can provide additional information to enhance diagnosis [51, 52].
- CT technologists should be aware of these applications of CT and continue learning about CT technical factors and dose optimization. In addition, technologists working in radiography, nuclear medicine, and radiation therapy, in particular, could benefit from learning more about CT scanning and certification.

References

1. Seeram, E. (2016). *Computed Tomography: Physical Principles, Clinical Applications, and Quality Control*. Philadelphia, PA: Saunders Elsevier.
2. Peterson, T.E. and Manning, H.C. (2009). Molecular imaging: 18F FDG PET and a whole lot more. *J. Nucl. Med. Technol.* 37 (3): 151–161. https://doi.org/10.2967/jnmt.109.062729.
3. Qiu, D. and Seeram, E. (2016). Does iterative reconstruction improve image quality and reduce dose in computed tomography? *Radiol. Open J.* 1 (2): 42–54. https://doi.org/10.17140/ROJ-1-108.
4. Bushong, S. (2017). Computed tomography. In: *Radiologic Science for Technologists*, 11e, 441–468. St Louis, MO: Mosby-Elsevier.
5. Wolbarst, A.B., Capasso, P., and Wyant, A.R. (2013). Computed tomography: superior contrast in three-dimensional x-ray attenuation maps. In: *Medical Imaging: Essentials for Physicians*, 191–233. Hoboken, NJ: Wiley.
6. Bushberg, J.T., Seibert, J.A., Leidholdt, E.M., and Boone, J.M. (2012). Computed tomography. In: *The Essential Physics of Medical Imaging*, 3e, 312–374. Philadelphia, PA: Lippincott Williams & Wilkins.
7. Herman, G.T. (1980). *Image Reconstruction from Projections*. New York: Academic Press.
8. Hsieh, J. (2008). Adaptive statistical iterative reconstruction. Whitepaper, GE Healthcare.
9. Hsieh, J., Nett, B., Yu, Z. et al. (2013). Recent advances in CT image reconstruction. *Curr. Radiol. Rep.* 1 (1): 39–51. https://doi.org/10.1007/s40134-012-0003-7.
10. Beister, M., Kolditz, D., and Kalender, W.A. (2012). Iterative reconstruction methods in x-ray CT. *Phys. Med.* 28 (2): 94–108. https://doi.org/10.1016/j.ejmp.2012.01.003.
11. Ehman, E.C., Yu, L., Manduca, A. et al. (2014). Methods for clinical evaluation of noise reduction techniques in abdominopelvic CT. *Radiographics* 34 (4): 849–862. https://doi.org/10.1148/rg344135128.

12. Seibert, J.A. (2014). Iterative reconstruction: how it works, how to apply it. *Pediatr. Radiol.* 44 (suppl 3): 431–439. https://doi.org/10.1007/s00247-014-3102-1.

13. Kaza, R.K., Platt, J.F., Goodsitt, M.M. et al. (2014). Emerging techniques for dose optimization in abdominal CT. *Radiographics* 34 (1): 4–17. https://doi.org/10.1148/rg.341135038.

14. Beck, T.J. (1996). CT technology overview: state of the art and future directions. In: *Syllabus: A Categorical Course in Physics—Technology Update and Quality Improvement of Diagnostic x-Ray Imaging Equipment* (eds. R.G. Gould and J.M. Boone), 161–172. Oak Brook, IL: Radiological Society of North America.

15. Fox, S.H. (1995). CT tube technology. In: *Medical CT and Ultrasound: Current Technology and Applications*, vol. 1995 (eds. L.W. Goldman and J.B. Fowlkes), 349–357. College Park, MD: American Association of Physicists in Medicine.

16. Homberg, R. and Koppel, R. (1997). An x-ray tube assembly with rotating-anode spiral groove bearing of the second generation. *Electromedica* 66: 65–66.

17. Shefer, E., Altman, A., Behling, R. et al. (2013). State of the art of CT detectors and sources: a literature review. *Curr. Radiol. Rep.* 1 (1): 76–91. https://doi.org/10.1007/s40134-012-0006.

18. Ulzheimer, S. and Kappler, S. (2017). Photon-counting detectors in clinical computed tomography. Siemens Healthineers website. https://health.siemens.com/ct_applications/somatomsessions/index.php/photon-counting-detectors-in-clinical-computed-tomography. Published January 12 (accessed 8 November 2017).

19. Xu, C. (2012). A segmented silicon strip detector for photon-counting spectral computed tomography. Doctoral thesis. AlbaNova Universitetscentrum. Kungliga Tekniska Högskolan, Stockholm.

20. Dalrymple, N.C., Prasad, S.R., El-Merhi, F.M., and Chintapalli, K.N. (2007). Price of isotropy in multidetector CT. *Radiographics* 27 (1): 49–62. https://doi.org/10.1148/rg.271065037.

21. IEC (1999). *Medical Electrical Equipment-60601 Part 2–44: Particular Requirements for the Safety of X-Ray Equipment for CT*. Geneva: International Electrotechnical Commission.

22. Pratx, G. and Xing, L. (2011). GPU computing in medical physics: a review. *Med. Phys.* 38 (5): 2685–2697. https://doi.org/10.1118/1.3578605.

23. Baxes, G.A. (1994). *Digital Image Processing: Principles and Applications*. New York: Wiley.

24. Seeram, E. and Seeram, D. (2008). Image postprocessing in digital radiology: a primer for technologists. *J. Med. Imag. Rad. Sci.* 39 (1): 23–41. https://doi.org/10.1016/j.jmir.2008.01.004.

25. Udupa, J. (2000). 3D imaging: principles and approaches. In: *3D Imaging in Medicine* (eds. J. Udupa and G. Herman), 1–74. Boca Raton, FL: CRC Press.

26. Silva, A.C., Wellnitz, C.V., and Hara, A.K. (2006). Three-dimensional virtual dissection at CT colonography: unraveling the colon to search for lesions. *Radiographics* 26 (6): 1669–1686. https://doi.org/10.1148/rg.266055199.

27. Pierce, L., Rosenberg, J., and Neustel, S. (2009). Trends in 3-D CT postprocessing. *Radiol. Technol.* 81 (1): 24–31.

28. Bibb, R. and Winder, J. (2010). A review of the issues surrounding 3D CT for medical modeling using rapid prototyping techniques. *Radiography* 16: 78–83. https://doi.org/10.1016/j.radi.2009.10.005.

29. Dalrymple, N.C., Prasad, S.R., Freckleton, M.W., and Chintapalli, K.N. (2005). Informatics in radiology (infoRAD): introduction to the language of three-dimensional imaging with multidetector CT. *Radiographics* 25 (5): 1409–1428. https://doi.org/10.1148/rg.255055044.

30. Gonzalez, R.C. and Woods, R.E. (2008). Image enhancement in the spatial domain. In: *Digital Image Processing*, 3e. Harlow: Prentice-Hall.

31. Kalender, W. (2005). *Computed Tomography Fundamentals, System Technology, Image Quality, Applications*. Erlangen: Publicis Corporate Publishing.

32. Hsieh, J. (2016). Image quality. In: *Computed Tomography: Physical Principles, Clinical Applications, and Quality Control* (ed. E. Seeram). Philadelphia, PA: Saunders Elsevier.

33. Seeram, E. (2018). *CT at a Glance*. Oxford: Wiley.

34. Barrett, J.F. and Keat, N. (2004). Artifacts in CT: recognition and avoidance. *Radiographics* 24 (6): 1679–1691. https://doi.org/10.1148/rg.246045065.

35. de Berrington, González, A., Mahesh, M., and Kim, K.-P. (2009). Projected cancer risks from computed tomographic scans performed in the United States in 2007. *Arch. Intern. Med.* 169 (22): 2071–2077. https://doi.org/10.1001/archinternmed.2009.440.

36. Van der Molen, A.J., Stoop, P., Prokop, M., and Geleijns, J. (2013). A national survey on radiation dose in CT in The Netherlands. *Insig. Imag.* 4 (3): 383–390. https://doi.org/10.1007/s13244-013-0253-9.

37. Mathews, J.D., Forsythe, A.V., Brady, Z. et al. (2013). Cancer risk in 680,000 people exposed to computed tomography scans in childhood or adolescence: data linkage study of 11 million Australians. *BMJ* 346: f2360. https://doi.org/10.1136/bmj.f2360.

38. Hricak, H., Brenner, D.J., Adelstein, S.J. et al. (2011). Managing radiation use in medical imaging: a multifaceted challenge. *Radiology* 258 (3): 889–905. https://doi.org/10.1148/radiol.10101157.

39. Toth, T., Ge, Z., and Daly, M.P. (2007). The influence of patient centering on CT dose and image noise. *Med. Phys.* 34 (7): 3093–3101. https://doi.org/10.1118/1.2748113.

40. Seeram, E. and Brennan, P.C. (2006). Diagnostic reference levels in radiology. *Radiol. Technol.* 77 (5): 373–384.

41. American College of Radiology (Revised 2013). ACR-AAPM practice parameter for diagnostic reference levels and achievable doses in medical x-ray imaging. https://www.acr.org/~/media/ACR/Documents/PGTS/guidelines/ReferenceLevelsDiagnostic_Xray.pdf?la=en (accessed 1 July 2017).

42. Seeram, E. (2014). Computed tomography dose optimization. *Radiol. Technol.* 85 (6): 655CT–671CT.

43. Valentin, J. and International Commission on Radiation Protection (2007). Managing patient dose in multi-detector computed tomography (MDCT). ICRP publication 102. *Ann. ICRP* 37 (1): 1–79.

44. U.S. Food and Drug Administration (Updated 1 April 2017). CFR-code of federal regulations-Title 21: Sec. 1020.33-Performance standards for ionizing radiation emitting products. https://www.accessdata.fda.gov/scripts/cdrh/cfdocs/cfCFR/CFRSearch.cfm?fr=1020.33 (accessed July 2017).

45. Government of Canada (2008). Safety code 35: safety procedures for installation, use and control of x-ray equipment in large medical radiological facilities. https://www.canada.ca/en/healthcanada/services/environmental-workplace-health/reports-publications/radiation/safety-code-35-safety-procedures-installation-use-control-equipment-large-medical-radiological-facilities-safety-code.html (accessed 8 November 2017).

46. Image gently website. http://www.imagegently.com (accessed 24 October 2020).

47. Image wisely website. http://www.imagewisely.org (accessed 24 October 2020).

48. Mather, R. (2007). *Aquilion ONE: Dynamic Volume CT*. Japan: Toshiba Medical Systems.

49. Kaza, R.K., Platt, J.F., Cohan, R.H. et al. (2012). Dual-energy CT with single- and dual-source scanners: current applications in evaluating the genitourinary tract. *Radiographics* 32 (2): 353–369. https://doi.org/10.1148/rg.322115065.

50. Mutic, S., Palta, J.R., Butker, E.K. et al. (2003). Quality assurance for CT simulators and CT simulation process. Report of the AAPM radiation therapy committee task group no 66. *Med. Phys.* 30: 2762–2792. https://doi.org/10.1118/1.1609271.

51. Patton, J.A. and Turkington, T.G. (2008). SPECT/CT physical principles and attenuation correction. *J. Nucl. Med. Technol.* 36 (1): 1–10. https://doi.org/10.2967/jnmt.107.046839.

52. Townsend, D.W. (2008). Positron emission tomography/computed tomography. *Semin. Nucl. Med.* 38 (3): 152–166. https://doi.org/10.1053/j.semnuclmed.2008.01.003.

53. Kim, M., Lee, J.M., Yoon, J.H. et al. (2014). Adaptive iterative dose reduction algorithm in CT: effect on image quality compared with filtered back projection in body phantoms of different sizes. *Korean J. Radiol.* 15 (2): 195–204.

SECTION 4

Continuous Quality Improvement

9

Fundamentals of quality control

INTRODUCTION

A significant and important requirement in imaging the patients is the principle of optimization, one of the fundamental radiation protection principles of the International Commission on Radiological Protection (ICRP). The optimization principle requires that radiation doses should be kept as low as reasonably achievable (ALARA) without compromising image quality. The quality of images obtained with low doses must be diagnostic. The ALARA philosophy is one of the major components of dose management. Furthermore, dose management is closely linked to the effectiveness of a *continuous quality improvement* (CQI) program introduced by The Joint Commission (TJC) in 1991. The CQI concept is an ongoing process, and that every employee plays a role in ensuring a quality product, and addresses a wide scope of issues relating to quality assurance (QA) and Quality Control (QC) designed to ensure optimal performance of personnel and equipment in the care and management of the patient.

The purpose of this chapter is to outline the essentials of QC rather that QA and CQI, since the principal activities of the technologist (and other qualified technical personnel such as medical physicists and clinical engineers) are related to the performance and ongoing evaluation of the equipment use to image patients. First, definitions of QA and QC are provided followed by a list of QC tools used for testing. Specifically, the parameters for QC testing, QC tests, and their tolerance limits for radiography, fluoroscopy, and computed tomography (CT) will be highlighted.

DEFINITIONS

The American Society for Quality defines QA and QC [1] as follows:

* *QA*: "The planned and systematic activities implemented in a quality system so that quality requirements for a product or service will be fulfilled."
* *QC*: "The observation techniques and activities used to fulfill requirements for quality."

These formal definitions can be applied to any vocation. In diagnostic radiology, QA and QC are integral components of the daily operations in radiography, fluoroscopy, mammography, and CT. QA and QC demand special attention in implementing the optimization principle of the ICRP. As summarized by Seeram [2], "QA is a term used to describe systems and procedures for assuring quality patient care. It deals specifically with quality assessment, continuing education, the usefulness of quality control procedures, and the assessment of outcomes. QA deals with the *administrative aspects* of patient care and quality outcomes. QC, on the other hand, is a component of QA and refers specifically to the monitoring of important variables that affect image quality and radiation dose. QC deals with the *technical aspects* (rather than administrative aspects) of equipment performance" [2]. Figure 9.1 illustrates the relationships among CQI, QA, and QC. QA is a subset of CQI, and QC is a subset of QA.

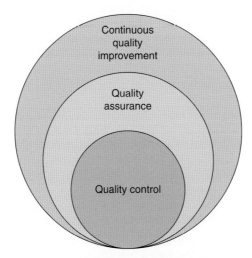

Figure 9.1　The relationships between CQI, QA, and QC. See text for further explanation.

Other organizations such as the National Council of Radiation Protection and Measurements (NCRP) [3], the American Association of Physicists in Medicine (AAPM) [4], and the American College of Radiology (ACR) [5], which specifically addresses accreditation issues, offer classic definitions and specific recommendations on QA and QC for diagnostic imaging. The interested reader should refer to these references for further information.

The purpose of CQI, QA, and QC is threefold:

1.   To ensure optimum image quality for the purpose of enhancing diagnosis.
2.   To optimize the radiation dose to patients and reduce the dose to personnel.
3.   To reduce costs to the institution.

Points 1 and 2 deal specifically with image quality and dose, and relate to the concept of dose optimization as described by the ICRP and requires that all personnel work within the ALARA philosophy, as mentioned above. Two *levels of optimization* are advocated by the ICRP:

•   the design and function of the x-ray imaging equipment and
•   imaging techniques and imaging protocols used during daily operation.

While the former examines the design and function of the equipment to meet current radiation protection standards, the latter deals with the procedural and operational practices during the conduct of the examination [6].

ESSENTIAL STEPS OF QC

The essential steps of QC are shown in Figure 9.2, and include acceptance testing, routine performance evaluation, and error correction. *Acceptance testing* means that all new imaging and image processing equipment meet the vendor's specifications as required by the department and operates efficiently in terms of dose output. It must also be conducted by a qualified individual, and not staff from the vendor. *Routine performance evaluation* refers to monitoring the components of the imaging system that affect dose and image quality. It includes QC tests that are performed daily, weekly, monthly, quarterly, and annually. The third step involves *error correction* which deals with the interpretation of the QC test results. In this regard, *tolerance limits* or *acceptance criteria* which have been previously established by objective and sometimes subject methods are used to check whether the component of the imaging system tested passes or fails the test. If the system fails the test, then it must be serviced to ensure that it will meet the tolerance limits or acceptance criteria. This is the fundamental tenet of error correction.

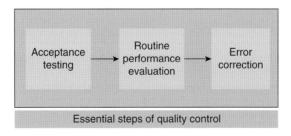

Figure 9.2   The essential steps of QC include acceptance testing, routine performance evaluation, and error correction.

QC RESPONSIBILITIES

Another principal tenet of CQI is that all personnel are involved in ensuring patient care and management, as well as the quality of the images produced. While this is true in radiology, personnel responsibilities for QC in particular have been described by the NCRP [3], AAPM [4], ACR [5] (in the United States), and by the Radiation Protection Bureau-Health Canada (RPB-HC) [7]. All of these organizations stress that a successful QC program requires the expertise of at least four classes of personnel, such as the radiologist, radiologic technologist, the medical physicist, in particular, a qualified medical physicist (QMP), and the imaging informatics professional (IIP). In summary of recommendations of the organizations listed above, the roles of each of these three professionals are as follows:

- First, as noted by Jones et al. [8], "the radiologist is the person ultimately responsible for the quality of the imaging practice. Therefore, the radiologist should participate in the design of the QC program and be available for consultation with the QC technologist and QMP when problems or questions arise. The radiologist should participate in the analysis process and in the implementation of corrective action when necessary."
- The QC technologist is one who is trained in QC and is responsible for conduct and operation of the QC program. Jones et al. [8] elaborates on the duties of the QC technologist as follows: "The QC technologist should ensure that all technologists involved in the radiography practice understand their responsibilities in the process. The QC technologist should manage the data collection and analysis, keep records, and perform other necessary administrative tasks. The QC technologist should perform quality control on the selected reasons for rejection and notify the QMP and radiologist of any problems or anomalies in the process. The QC technologist should work with the QMP to implement suggestions for correcting malfunctioning equipment and practice problems."
- The ACR [9] provides an overview statement on the role of the QMP and states that "the QMP is uniquely qualified to perform certain tests and then analyze the data to determine which sets of specifications are relevant to a particular imaging problem. The QMP is able to bridge the gap between the technical aspects and clinical image quality of the system. The QMP testing allows the QMP to recognize equipment failures before they unacceptably degrade clinical images. The QMP can also perform tests to determine if imaging irregularities can be attributed to procedural or equipment errors."
- Additionally, the ACR, AAPM, and Society for Imaging Informatics in Medicine (SIIM) in their technical standard for electronic practice of medical imaging have identified the *IIP*, since this individual plays an integral role in the digital infrastructure of imaging departments. The IIP should be qualified in areas of computer networking infrastructure, databases, data entry, and management systems and have qualifications in a wide range of computer operating systems, internet protocols, and systems related to picture archiving and communication systems (PACS), radiology information systems (RIS), and hospital information systems (HIS), and so forth.

STEPS IN CONDUCTING A QC TEST

Conducting QC tests for the evaluation of equipment performance requires the use of a defined set of rules for solving a problem as illustrated in the flowchart in Figure 9.3. The steps in performing a QC test include:

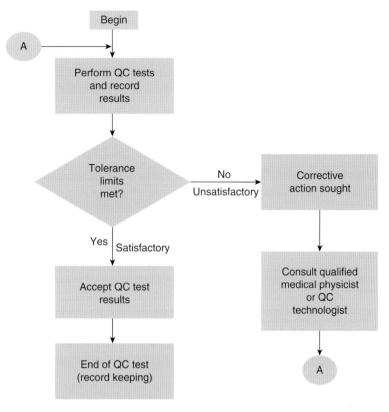

Figure 9.3 Conducting QC tests for the evaluation of equipment performance requires the use of a defined set of rules for solving a problem as illustrated in the flowchart.

1. Begin the test procedure (after gathering the tools needed to perform the test).
2. Conduct the test and document the results.
3. Interpret the results.
4. If the tolerance limits have been met, then accept the results and begin another test. The equipment passes the test.
5. If the results have not been met, the equipment fails the test. Seek corrective action.
6. Consult a QMP and/or a QC technologist. The IIP may also have to be consulted if it falls within the domain of informatics (information technology).
7. After consultation, repeat the test until tolerance limits have been met.
8. It is mandatory that records of all QC tests be kept, not only to examine trends, but importantly for accreditation purposes.

THE TOLERANCE LIMIT OR ACCEPTANCE CRITERIA

Evaluation of the results of QC tests requires established acceptance criteria or tolerance limits. These criteria or limits have been classified as *quantitative* (established by objective means) as well as *qualitative* (established by subjective means) as illustrated in Figure 9.4.

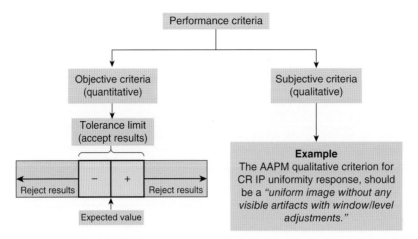

Figure 9.4 Evaluation of the results of QC tests require established acceptance criteria or tolerance limits. These criteria or limits have been classified as *quantitative* (established by objective means) as well as *qualitative* (established by subjective means). See text for further explanation.

If the results of a QC test fall within the tolerance limit, then the test results are acceptable. On the other hand, if the results exceed the tolerance limits, the results indicate that the equipment performance is unacceptable and must be serviced immediately. In Figure 9.4, the expected value is also shown. This means that if a QC test, for example, examined kV accuracy, and the technologist selected 100 kV as the test kV, then the results should be 100 kV (expected value) if the machine is performing accurately. The results obtained after this test is 90 kV. Should the technologist accept this result? (See the third bullet in the following list.)

Examples of *quantitative limits* are:

- The tolerance limit for collimation of the x-ray beam QC test should be ±2% of the source-to-image receptor distance (SID) [10].
- For retake/reject analysis in digital radiography, the AAPM recommends that "a lower threshold of 5% be used as a threshold for investigation and possible corrective action unless clinical data indicate this threshold should be lower" [8].
- For kV calibration QC test, the measured kV should be within 10% of the indicated kV [10].

Examples of *qualitative criteria* are:

- For *erasure thoroughness of the* CR *imaging plate (IP)* QC test, the criterion is the absence of a ghost image of the step wedge from the first exposure in the re-exposed image.
- For the *dark noise* (level of noise present in the system) QC test in digital radiography, the acceptable criterion is uniform image without artifacts.

Other limits will be highlighted further in the section "Performance Criteria/Tolerance Limits for Common QC Tests".

PARAMETERS FOR QC MONITORING

The parameters for QC testing in digital radiography generally relate to major components of the imaging equipment, including electronic display devices and to the integrity of protective equipment, etc. It is not within the scope of this chapter to outline all the system parameters that are subject to QC procedures; however, the following parameters for QC testing are noteworthy because they are commonplace.

Major parameters of imaging systems

Imaging systems refer to film-screen radiography (FSR), CR, flat-panel digital radiography (FPDR), digital fluoroscopy (DF), and CT. FSR and image intensifier-based DF have been replaced almost totally by digital radiology modalities (CR, FPDR, and DF). Generally, a few of the most common parameters for FSR, CR, FPDR, fluoroscopy, and CT include:

- Equipment warm-up and overall visual inspection of system components to ensure cleanliness and integrity of performance, such as system movements allowed.
- Retake analysis.
- Filtration, collimation, and focal spot size.
- kV and timer accuracy.
- Exposure linearity and reproducibility.
- Protective apparel.
- Exposure index (EI) and dynamic range.
- Dark noise, IP uniformity, spatial accuracy, erasure thoroughness.
- Entrance skin exposure rate, Automatic intensity control.
- Electronic display performance.
- CT number accuracy, CT noise, CT uniformity, calibration of the CT number.
- CT spatial resolution and CT low contrast detectability.
- CT laser light accuracy.
- CT radiation dose.

QC TESTING FREQUENCY

Testing frequency refers to how often a QC test should be performed. Today, QC testing frequencies are divided into daily, weekly, monthly, quarterly, and annually, as classified by various organizations such as the ACR [5, 9], AAPM [4, 9, 11], and RPB-HC [7]. The following are a few tests for CR, FPDR, and fluoroscopy, and the frequencies with which they should be conducted as recommended by RPB-HC [7].

QC tests have been organized into ones that the technologist performs.

- *Daily tests*: Equipment warm-up, equipment conditions, and visual assessment of electronic display devices.
- *Weekly tests*: Visual inspection of cleanliness of imaging systems.
- *Monthly tests*: Electronic device display performance, and retake analysis for FSR, CR, and FPDR systems.

- *Quarterly tests*: Collimation operation, interlocks. Furthermore, protective devices should be evaluated quarterly.
- *Annual tests*: Radiation output reproducibility, radiation beam linearity, x-ray beam filtration, automatic exposure control (AEC), collimation, and grid performance.

For CT specifically, the ACR [9] recommends the following tests (for technologists) and their minimum frequencies:

- *Daily tests*: Water CT number and standard deviation, and artifact evaluation.
- *Weekly tests*: Wet laser printer QC.
- *Monthly tests*: Visual checklist, dry laser printer QC, and gray level performance of the CT scanner acquisition display monitors.

TOOLS FOR QC TESTING

The tools for QC testing range from *simple tools* to more *complex tools* used to check the performance of the imaging system components that play a role in affecting the dose to the patient as well as influencing image quality. While simple tools include approved screen-cleaning and cloths, film-screen contact test tool, dosimeters, aluminum filters, multiple sheets of tissue equivalent attenuator, a step-wedge, x-ray beam alignment tool, and so forth, complex tools include the Society of Motion Picture and Television Engineers (SMPTE) test pattern, high-contrast resolution line pair phantoms (up to 5 lp/mm), low-contrast phantoms, and vendor-recommended photostimulable phosphor (PSP) phantom, etc.

For CT QC, special equipment and phantoms are available such as image performance phantoms, geometric phantoms, and quantitative dosimetry phantoms and instrumentation [9, 12].

An important tool that is now commonplace in digital radiography and CT is the *SMPTE test pattern* shown in Figure 9.5. The pattern is used to evaluate display devices in the digital radiology department, including the CT department. As described by the ACR, there are several components that are used to test the display quality, as shown in Figure 9.5. "The first component is a rectangular collection of square patches of different gray levels ranging from 0 to 100% in increments of 10%. The second component is a pair of square gray level patches, each with a smaller patch of slightly different gray level inside: one is a 0 patch with a 5% patch inside, and the other is a 100% patch with a 95% patch inside. These are referred to as the 0/5% patch and the 95/100% patch, respectively" [9]. This pattern can be used to test geometric distortions, reflection, luminance response, display resolution, and display noise, In particular, "the most common is the observation of 5 and 95% luminance patches. This helps to point out any gross deviations in luminance adjustments" [10].

THE FORMAT OF A QC TEST

Figure 9.3 shows a flowchart of a typical approach to conducting a QC test. In general, QC tests must be done systematically in order to provide accurate results. While the format of QC tests will differ from country to country and from institution to institution, the ACR(9) provides a format as follows:

- Objective
- Frequency
- Required Equipment
- Test Procedure
- Data Interpretation and Corrective Action

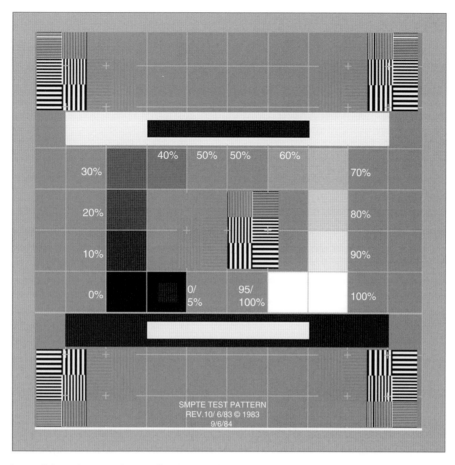

Figure 9.5 A useful tool to evaluate display performance in digital radiography and CT is the SMPTE test pattern.

PERFORMANCE CRITERIA/TOLERANCE LIMITS FOR COMMON QC TESTS

It is not within the scope of this chapter to list the limits for all imaging modalities, and therefore only the more common ones will be highlighted for radiography, fluoroscopy, and CT. These limits are the range of values that are deemed acceptable for equipment components that have passed the tests. It is important to note, however, that the limits listed below are not internationally accepted limits. Therefore, technologists must consult the QC requirements of their respective countries. The limits below are examples from the NCRP [3], ACR [4], AAPM [5], and RPB-HC [7].

Radiography

Visual inspection
The purpose of visual inspection is to examine all aspects of the equipment to ensure that they will provide for comfort and safety of both patients and personnel during the examination.

- Some items are inspected on a daily basis; others will require annual inspection.
- The tolerance limits are qualitative. All problems and potential problems must be reported to the manager and clinical engineer-medical physicist who should address the means to rectify problems that pose a danger to patients and personnel.

Filtration

- The total filtration for all radiographic units is 2.5 mm a (Al).
- The frequency of filtration test is annually.
- The tolerance limit for filtration depends on the kV used. For example, RPB-HC [7] specifies the following:
  - 70 kV: 2.5 mm Al
  - 90 kV: 3.2 mm Al
  - 120 kV: 4.3 mm Al

Collimation

The purpose of the collimation QC test is to check the alignment of the light field of the collimator and the radiation field shaped by the collimator. These two fields must be in perfect alignment. Automatic collimation (positive beam limitation, PBL) should also be tested to ensure that the x-ray field size is not larger than the size of the image receptor.

- The tolerance limit for light field and x-ray field alignment is such that the misalignment must not be greater than ±2% of the SID. For PBL systems, the misalignment must not be greater than ±3% of the SID.

Focal spot size

QC test should be performed only during the acceptance testing stage, or it can be checked annually as well.

- The measured size may be 50% greater than the stated size and still be within acceptable limits. Therefore, for a 0.3×0.3 mm focal spot size, 0.45×0.65 mm can be tolerated. For a 1.0×1.0 mm size, 1.4×2.0 mm is acceptable. For a 2.0×2.0 mm, 2.6×2.7 is acceptable. If these sizes are greater, then the x-ray tube should be changed.

kV accuracy

The kV affects both the dose the patient receives and the image contrast. Low kV means greater contrast but higher patient dose resulting from the predominance of the photoelectric absorption.

- The purpose of the kV QC test is to check the accuracy of the kV. The technologist wants to find out whether the measured kV is the same as that selected on the control panel for the examination.
- Test should be performed annually.
- Tolerance limit is that the measured kV should be within 10% of the indicated kV set on the control panel.

Exposure timer accuracy

The tolerance limits are as follows:

For manual timers:

- Accuracy should be within 5% of the time set on the unit for times greater than 10 milliseconds (ms).
- For exposure times of 10 ms or less, an accuracy of 20% is acceptable.

- For AEC for digital systems, "the performance of the AEC must be assessed according to the manufacturer's procedures and must be within the manufacturer's specifications. . ..compliance is checked by ensuring that the ratio of the highest to the lowest measured value is less than or equal to 1.2 or within the manufacturer's specifications" [9].

Exposure linearity

The same mAs values for different combinations of mA and time settings that produce the same exposure output is referred to as the exposure linearity.

- Purpose of the exposure linearity QC test is to check that the same exposure output is measured for different combinations of mA and time that produce the same mAs.
- This test should be done once a year.
- The tolerance limit for this test is that the linearity should be within 10% for adjacent mA settings. A calibrated dosimeter must be used to measure radiation output [10].

Exposure uniformity

When the same mA, time, and kV values are used repeatedly, the exposure output for each exposure should be the same.

- This test should be done annually.
- The tolerance limit is that the output exposure should be reproducible to within 5% [10].

Exposure index, dynamic range, and noise, spatial resolution, and contrast detectability

It is generally recommended that these parameters be evaluated using the vendor's recommended test procedures and that the results must be within the vendor's established limits. Technologists and the QMP must consult the literature provided by vendors for their respective digital imaging systems.

Electronic display performance

The AAPM [13] identifies four categories of displays, namely, diagnostic displays, modality displays, clinical specialty displays, and the electronic health record (EHR) displays. All these display devices are subject to performance evaluations, and the AAPM Task Group (TG) Report 270 [13] provides both qualitative and quantitative criteria for performance. Furthermore, this report introduces and describes *new test patterns* to be used for display performance, compared to the older test patterns, the SMPTE and TG-18 patterns. These patterns are used to evaluate geometric distortion, reflection, luminance response, display resolution, noise, veiling glare, and chromaticity. It is not within the scope of this chapter to describe each of these, and therefore the interested reader may refer to Bushong [10] for detailed descriptions.

For the evaluation of gray level performance of the acquisition display characteristics, the ACR [9] states that:

The visual impression should indicate an even progression of gray levels around the "ring" of gray level patches. Verify the following: (i) the 5% patch can be distinguished in the 0/5% patch; (ii) the 95% patch can be distinguished in the 95/100% patch; and (iii) all the gray level steps around the ring of gray levels are distinct from adjacent steps (note that there are two adjacent squares that are both labelled as 50% which should appear to be equivalent). If these conditions are not met, do not adjust the display window width/level in an effort to correct the problem. Corrective action for the monitor is needed.

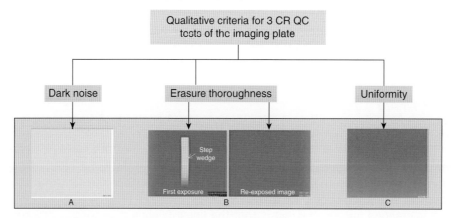

Figure 9.6   Qualitative acceptance criteria for three QC tests of the CR IP, dark noise, erasure thoroughness, and uniformity.

Computed radiography: qualitative acceptance criteria – three examples

The AAPM [11] in Report 93-*Acceptance Testing and Quality Control of Photostimulable Storage Phosphor Imaging Systems* provides both quantitative and qualitative criteria for CR QC parameters. Two of these, dark noise and erasure thoroughness, were mentioned earlier in this chapter. The other two are the CR IP uniformity and spatial accuracy. In summary, the criteria are as follows for three parameters:

* *Dark noise*: Uniform image without artifacts (Figure 9.6a).
* *Erasure thoroughness*: The absence of a ghost image of the step wedge from the first exposure to the re-exposed image (Figure 9.6b).
* *Uniformity*: Uniform image without artifacts (Figure 9.6c).

Fluoroscopy

Fluoroscopy has evolved from image intensifier-based DF to DF using the flat-panel digital detector. One of the major concerns in fluoroscopic examinations is that the patient dose can be high [10]. In particular, the *entrance skin dose* (ESD) is important because of the potential of causing skin erythema. The ESD should always be measured using a calibrated dosimeter and is carried out by a QMP. The QC test result should be such that the ESD rate should not exceed 100 mGy/minute (10 R/min) [10].

In addition to the ESD measurement, there are several other QC tests including filtration, focal spot size, kV accuracy, mA linearity, exposure reproducibility, grid uniformity and alignment, automatic brightness control, resolution (spatial and contrast), and the television monitor performance. It is not within the scope of this chapter to describe all the fluoroscopic parameters that require QC monitoring. It is important to realize, however, that certain tests should be carried out daily, weekly, monthly, and annually. Daily tests, for example, include equipment warm-up, system movements, and overall visual assessment of electronic display devices. While weekly tests include visual inspection of cleanliness of the system components, monthly tests focus on collimation operation, interlocks, table movements, compression devices operation, fluoroscopic cumulative timer operation, and protective devices. Examples of annually tests are radiation output reproducibility and linearity, filtration, AEC, x-ray field and light field alignment and collimation, grid performance, dynamic range, spatial resolution, contrast detectability, automatic intensity control, image lag, integrity of protective equipment, and so forth [9]. These tests in fluoroscopy are often conducted by the QMP.

Integrity of protective equipment refers to all personnel protective equipment. These can be examined using both radiography and fluoroscopy to ensure they offer the protective requirements needed. For example, for lead aprons, where "the total defective area is greater than 670 mm^2 are not acceptable. Personnel protective equipment having a defect in the vicinity of the thyroid or the reproductive organs which is larger than the equivalent of a 5 mm diameter circle must not be used. . ..All protective equipment, when not in use, should be stored in accordance with the manufacturers' recommendations" [7].

REPEAT IMAGE ANALYSIS

A *repeat image analysis* (RIA) has its origins in FSR and was referred to as a *reject analysis program* (RAP). RAP became an integral component of FSR QC program. Since the program is related to film, it was also referred to as a *repeat/reject film analysis*. The central activity in a repeat film analysis is a careful and systematic assessment of the reasons why films had to be repeated or why they have been rejected. In summary:

- The benefits of a repeat film analysis are to improve the efficiency of the examination, to reduce the costs associated with films and processing, and to minimize the dose to patients from repeat exposures.
- The repeat film analysis includes collecting and sorting rejected films into various categories that identify the reasons films were discarded. Examples of these categories are poor positioning, poor density and contrast, blurring from patient motion, and the presence of artifacts and processing errors.
- The repeat rate can be calculated knowing the total number of films used during the period of the study and the total number of patients involved.
- The repeat rate (%) = number of repeated films/total number of films × 100.
- The overall repeat rate should be less than 2% as should the rate for each category [10]. When repeat rates exceed these limits, corrective action is required.

Corrective action/Reasons for rejection

The AAPM TG 151 published a report on "Ongoing Quality Control in Digital Radiography" [9], with the goal of providing additional guidance on rejected image analysis, exposure analysis, and artifact identification, as part of the QC process. This section will focus only on the continued need for RIA and corrective action.

The motivation for the continued need for RIA is based on manual collection of data for the RAP and other shortcomings such as "including lack of RT compliance, intentional circumvention of the program, accidental deletion of data, and false negative or false positive results" [9]. To solve these problems, other methods were needed such as server-based RAP "that automatically collect, parse, and analyze data from many different acquisition systems spread throughout an institution" [9]. Furthermore, in digital radiography, AAPM Report TG-151 states that "the rejected image rate in its simplest form can be calculated as the ratio of the number of rejected images to the total number of images acquired" [9].

- *Corrective action*: In digital radiography, the literature reports that rejected image rates range from 4 to 8% [14–16]. With this in mind, the AAPM TG-151 recommends that "8% be used as a target for overall rejected image rate, and 10% as a threshold for investigation and possible corrective action" [9]. "It has been proposed that there is a baseline repeat rate of 5%, below which radiographic quality is sacrificed and further reduction is not cost-effective" [9].
- *Standardized reasons for rejection*: The AAPM TG-151 notes that these reasons should include positioning, exposure error, grid error, system error, artifact, patient motion, test images, study canceled, and others.

COMPUTED TOMOGRAPHY QC TESTS FOR TECHNOLOGISTS

The CT scanner is a complex medical device, and as such it is subject to routine performance evaluation of a wide range of technical parameters. Examples of these parameters include equipment warm-up, visual inspection and cleanliness of the system, visual assessment of electronic display devices, CT number accuracy, image noise, uniformity, section thickness, linearity, patient support movements, spatial resolution, low-contrast detectability, laser light accuracy, gantry-tilt accuracy, patient dose, etc.

A number of organizations, such as the AAPM, the ACR, RBP-HC, and the IAEA (International Atomic Energy Agency), have recommended that specific QC tests be done daily, weekly, monthly, semi-annually, and annually. They have also recommended that certain tests be done by technologists and others be done by QMPs. The ACR, in their CT QC manual, outlines responsibilities for the supervising radiologist, including a section describing the leadership role of the radiologist in a CT QC program. One such important role is that "the radiologist is ultimately responsible for the quality of images produced under their direction and bears ultimate responsibility for both proper QC testing and QA procedures in CT" [9]. Furthermore, the ACR recommends that the tests done by a QMP, for example, include spatial resolution, low-contrast performance, CT number accuracy and uniformity, CT dosimetry, and CT scanner display calibration, all of which should be done annually.

QC tests that are recommended by the ACR and the IAEA to be conducted by the technologist/radiographer are listed in Table 9.1. In this section, only those tests recommended by the ACR for technologists will be highlighted.

The ACR CT accreditation phantom

The ACR suggests that the ACR CT accreditation phantom be used to perform required CT QC tests. A general schematic of the phantom is shown in Figure 9.7. The phantom consists of four modules, each of which is designed to measure specific parameters, as shown. Additionally, the head and foot ends of the phantom are also labeled, to guide set-up procedures during QC testing. The ACR provides an example of how to conduct the QC test for "Water CT Number and Standard Deviation (Noise)" using the ACR CT QC phantom [9] as outlined in Table 9.2.

Table 9.1 QC tests recommended by the ACR and the IAEA, to be done by technologists/radiographers.

ACR	IAEA
1. Water CT number and standard deviation (D)	1. CT alignment lights
2. Artifact evaluation (D)	2. SPR accuracy
3. Wet laser printer QC (W)	3. CT number accuracy
4. Visual checklist (M)	4. CT image noise
5. Dry laser printer QC (M)	5. CT image uniformity
6. Gray level performance of the CT scanner	6. CT image artifact assessment
7. Acquisition display monitors (M)	7. Image display and printing

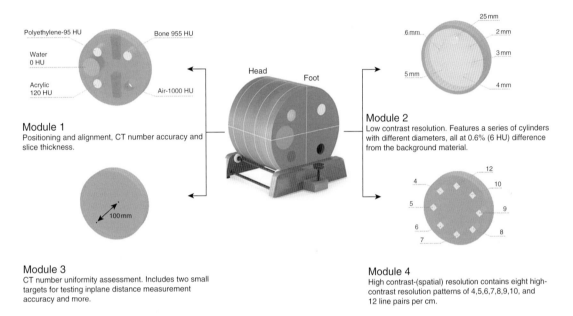

Module 1
Positioning and alignment, CT number accuracy and slice thickness.

Module 2
Low contrast resolution. Features a series of cylinders with different diameters, all at 0.6% (6 HU) difference from the background material.

Module 3
CT number uniformity assessment. Includes two small targets for testing inplane distance measurement accuracy and more.

Module 4
High contrast-(spatial) resolution contains eight high-contrast resolution patterns of 4,5,6,7,8,9,10, and 12 line pairs per cm.

Figure 9.7 A general schematic of the ACR CT QC accreditation phantom. The phantom consists of four modules, each of which is designed to measure specific parameters, as illustrated. See text for further explanation. *Source*: Images Courtesy of Gammex, Sun Nuclear Corporation.

The ACR action limits for tests done by technologists

As shown in Table 9.1, there are six QC tests to be conducted by technologists, but only two action limits will be provided here, namely, water CT number and standard deviation (daily frequency) and the gray level performance of the CT scanner. The interested reader should refer to the ACR CT QC Manual [9].

- *Water CT number and standard deviation*
  The QMP, after consulting the manufacturer's specifications, should provide limit criteria for water mean and standard deviation. Typically, mean values for water fall within 0+/−3 HU; however, they must be within 0±5 HU or as the manufacturer specifies. Limit criteria for the noise (standard deviation) values are primarily determined by the scan technique (radiation).

- *Gray level of CT scanner acquisition display monitors*

Table 9.2 An example of a QC test format.

Water CT number and standard deviation (noise)	
Objective	To ensure that the calibration of CT numbers relative to water remains within acceptable limits and that quantum noise and electronic system noise do not increase. Excessive image noise degrades low-contrast detectability and can be a symptom of other system problems.
Frequency	Daily
Required equipment	The water phantom provided by the scanner manufacturer or the ACR CT phantom. Data can be recorded on the Data Form for Daily CT Equipment Quality Control
Test procedure	1. Warm up the scanner's x-ray tube according to manufacturer recommendations. 2. Perform calibration scans (often called air-calibration scans) according to scanner manufacturer recommendations. 3. Place the QC phantom on the holder device provided. Center the phantom at the isocenter of the scanner using the laser alignment lights of the scanner and the alignment marks on the phantom surface. 4. Set up a scan of the QC phantom using the scanner's daily QC scan parameter settings. It is strongly recommended that the QC scan protocols be preprogrammed for consistency. Usually, these scan protocols will follow the parameter settings recommended by the scanner manufacturer. Water mean and standard deviation values must be monitored in either the axial or helical scan mode and may be monitored in both modes; that is, the QMP should assist the QC technologist to establish (and ideally preprogram) the desired scan in one of these modes. If the QMP desires, then they can assist the QC technologist in establishing (and again, ideally preprogram) the desired scan for the other mode, which will typically be performed less frequently
Data interpretation and corrective action	1. If a group of images were obtained on a multislice CT scanner, for example, then select an image from the central portion of the group to analyze. Place a region-of-interest (ROI) at the center of the image. If the size of this ROI is not specified by the scanner manufacturer, use an area around $400\,mm^2$. Record the values reported for the water mean and standard deviation, which can be recorded on the data form. 2. Repeat Steps 1 and 2 for image(s) acquired in the second scan mode (if performed). 3. The QMP, after consulting the manufacturer's specifications, should provide limit criteria for water mean and standard deviation. Typically, mean values for water fall within $0\pm3\,HU$; however, they must be within $0\pm5\,HU$ or as the manufacturer specifies. Limit criteria for the noise (standard deviation) values are primarily determined by the scan technique (radiation dose) used to acquire the images. If the QMP elects to use the manufacturer's specified standard deviation as the limit criteria, the scan technique must be identical to the manufacturer's recommendation (including reconstructed image thickness and reconstruction kernel or filter). 4. If the ACR CT phantom is used as the QC phantom, the water value should be $0\pm5\,HU$, but must be $0\pm7\,HU$. Note that the baseline value might be different on some scanners and should be established by the QMP. The QMP may establish limit criteria for noise (standard deviation) for either axial or helical modes (or both) after consulting manufacturer's recommendations. Due to scanner and setup fluctuations, it may be advisable to perform a 10-day (or more) average of standard deviation data when establishing baselines. 5. If either the mean CT number or the noise (standard deviation) is not within the criteria established by the QMP, then the phantom, phantom positioning, phantom image used, ROI placement, and protocol used should be double checked. Additionally, air calibrations (if recommended by the manufacturer) should be run. The test should then be repeated. If the test is still failing, consult the QMP for guidance. The QMP should assist in determining whether or not service should be contacted, and, if necessary, if the service should be done prior to clinical imaging.

Source: Based on from the ACR [9].

The visual impression should indicate an even progression of gray levels around the "ring" of gray level patches. Verify the following: a) the 5% patch can be distinguished in the 0/5% patch; b) the 95% patch can be distinguished in the 95/100% patch; and c) all the gray level steps around the ring of gray levels are distinct from adjacent steps (note that there are two adjacent squares that are both labelled as 50% which should appear to be equivalent). If these conditions are not met, do not adjust the display window width/level in an effort to correct the problem. Corrective action for the monitor is needed.

Artifact evaluation

As shown in Table 9.1, the ACR also assigns the task of artifact evaluation to the technologist to be done on a daily basis. The ACR CT phantom may be used or the vendor's water phantom. The overall goal of this test is to "identify and correct artifacts in images of a uniform test phantom before they become severe enough to be detected in patient images" [9].

Artifacts can arise from a number of different sources leading to streak artifacts, shading artifacts, and ring artifacts, as illustrated in Figure 9.8. While streaks are created from undersampling, partial volume averaging, patient motion, metal, beam hardening, noise, and mechanical failure, shading artifacts arise from partial volume averaging, beam hardening, for example. Finally, ring artifacts arise from bad detector channels in third-generation CT scanners. Additional artifacts are illustrated in the ACR CT QC manual [9]. Other sources, such as Seeram [17] and Kofler [18], provide further detailed descriptions, as well as images of these artifacts.

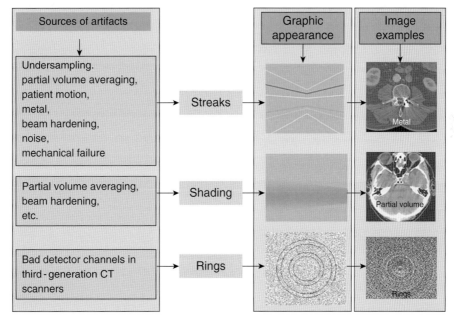

Figure 9.8 Artifacts can arise from a number of different sources leading to streak artifacts, shading artifacts, and ring artifacts. See text for further explanation. *Source*: From Seeram [12], reproduced with permission. © 2018, John Wiley & Sons.

References

1. American Society for Quality (2020). *Definitions of Quality Assurance and Quality Control*. https://asq.org/quality-resources/quality-glossary (accessed June 2020).
2. Seeram, E. (2019). *Digital Radiography: Physical Principles and Quality Control*, 2e. Singapore: Springer Nature Singapore Pte Ltd.
3. National Council on Radiation Protection and Measurements (NCRP) (1988). Quality Assurance for Diagnostic Imaging. Bethesda, MD: NCRP. *NCRP Report 99*.
4. American Association of Physicists in Medicine (AAPM) (2002). Quality Control in Diagnostic Radiology. Madison, WI: Medical Physics. *Report 74*.
5. American College of Radiology, (ACR) (2006). *ACR Technical Standard for Diagnostic Medical Physics Performance Monitoring of Radiographic and Fluoroscopic Equipment*, 1139–1142. Reston, VA: ACR.
6. Seeram, E. and Brennan, P. (2017). *Radiation Protection in Diagnostic X-Ray Imaging*, 2017. Burlington, MA: Jones and Bartlett Learning.
7. Radiation Protection Bureau-Health Canada (RPB-HC) (2008). Radiation Protection in Radiology-Large Facilities. Ottawa: Minister of Health. *Safety Code-35*.
8. Jones, A.K., Heintz, P., Geiser, W. et al. (2015). Ongoing quality control in digital radiography: report of AAPM Imaging Physics Committee Task Group 151. *Med. Phys.* 42 (11): 6658–6670.
9. American College of Radiology, (ACR) (2017). *2017 CT Quality Control Manual. Qualified Medical Physicist Section*, 53–86. Reston, VA: ACR.
10. Bushong, S. (2017). *Radiologic Science for Technologists*, 11e. Elsevier: St Louis, MO.
11. American Association of Physicists in Medicine (AAPM) (2006). Acceptance Testing and Quality Control of Photostimulable Storage Phosphor Imaging Systems. Madison, WI: Medical Physics. *Report 93*.
12. Seeram, E. (2018). *CT at a Glance*. Hoboken, NJ: Wiley.
13. American Association of Physicists in Medicine (AAPM) (2019). *Display QA-TG Report 270*. Alexandria, VG: AAPM.
14. Nol, J., Isouard, G., and Mirecki, J. (2006). Digital repeat analysis; setup and operation. *J. Digit. Imag.* 19: 159–166.
15. Peer, S., Peer, R., Walcher, M. et al. (1999). Comparative reject analysis in conventional film-screen and digital storage phosphor radiography. *Eur. Radiol.* 9: 1693–1696.
16. Weatherburn, G.C., Bryan, S., and West, M. (1999). A comparison of image reject rates when using film, hard copy computed radiography and soft copy images on picture archiving and communication systems (PACS) workstations. *Br. J. Radiol.* 72: 653–660.
17. Seeram, E. (2016). *Computed Tomography: Physical Principles, Clinical Applications, and Quality Control*, 5e. St Louis, MO: Elsevier.
18. Kofler JM. (2018). *Identifying image artifacts, their causes, and how to fix them; computed tomography*. AAPM Annual General Meeting 2018. AAPM.

SECTION 5
PACS and Imaging Informatics

10

PACS and imaging informatics at a glance

INTRODUCTION

The term imaging informatics (II) refers to the application of information technology (IT) concepts to diagnostic imaging modalities such as digital radiography (DR) and digital fluoroscopy (DF), computed tomography (CT), magnetic resonance imaging (MRI), and diagnostic medical sonography (DMS). Furthermore, since radiation therapy (RT) and nuclear medicine (NM) incorporate CT into their clinical, education, and research environments, they are also included in the II framework. Additionally, since medical imaging and RT are integral components of healthcare, II includes aspects of what has been referred to as healthcare informatics. II is now a new subdiscipline in medical imaging and RT.

A Comprehensive Guide to Radiographic Sciences and Technology, First Edition. Euclid Seeram.
© 2021 John Wiley & Sons Ltd. Published 2021 by John Wiley & Sons Ltd.

In 1997, Kulikowski et al. [1] suggested that the tasks performed by computers in the radiology department provided the basis for II. Specifically, these tasks relate to digital image acquisition, digital image processing and image display, image storage and archiving, computer networking, and image transmission. The result of the active use of these technologies is the production of very large amounts of digital data including image and text data. This situation posed a challenge of how to effectively handle these large data sets in terms of archiving, storage, and communicating information from such digital data. The solution was to develop a picture archiving and communication system (PACS). PACS is now an important and significant tool in the digital radiology department.

The purpose of this chapter is to present a broad overview of the major components and technologies characteristic of PACS. Furthermore, the chapter will outline the basics of II and briefly explain the emerging trends in II, as a necessary foundation needed for the further study of II.

PACS CHARACTERISTIC FEATURES

Definition

The literature provides several definitions of PACS; however, the following definition is simple and meaningful and meets the overall goal of this book. Samei et al. [2] state that PACS is:

. . ..a comprehensive computer system that is responsible for the electronic storage and distribution of medical images in the medical enterprise. The system is highly integrated with digital acquisition and display devices and is often related closely to other medical information systems, such as the Radiology Information System (RIS) or Hospital Information System (HIS).

Core technical components

The functional organization of the major system components of a typical PACS is illustrated in Figure 10.1, and include image acquisition modalities, such as DR, DF, CT, MRI, DMS, and NM; acquire digital images that are subsequently sent to the PACS host computer; and special devices called as interfaces are responsible for connecting acquisition devices, information systems, and the world wide web to the PACS host computer. Additionally, image display workstations are essential components all of which are connected and linked to the hospital information system (HIS) and the radiology information system (RIS), through digital communication networks.

The central component of the system is the PACS "high-end" host computer or server. After images are acquired (image acquisition), they are sent to the to the host computer. Furthermore, patient data such as demographics, for example, are sent from the information systems (HIS/RIS) to the host computer which has a database server as well as an archive system. PACS archiving devices include laser optical disks, a redundant array of independent disks (RAID), and magnetic tapes.

Images are displayed on the monitors of workstations for the purpose of image interpretation. There are a number of classes of workstations depending on how they are used. Radiologists must have *high-resolution diagnostic workstations* that allow them to interpret images and provide a diagnosis. Technologists often use *review workstations* for general assessment of image quality

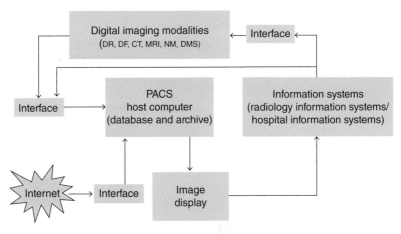

Figure 10.1   The functional organization of the major system components of a typical PACS.

before the images are sent to the PACS. These workstations feature digital postprocessing software to allow users to manipulate images for the purpose of enhancing diagnosis. For example, image compression can be used to reduce storage space and decrease image transmission times.

There are additional features of PACS which enable effective and efficient function.

One such notable feature is the use of industry healthcare standards for the communication of both images and text data. While image communications require the use of the Digital Imaging and Communications in Medicine (DICOM) standard, text communications make use of Health Level-7 (HL-7).

While DICOM is concerned primarily with images from the digital image acquisition modalities, HL-7 is concerned mainly with textual information from the HIS and RIS. Since the PACS contain confidential patient data and information, it is essential that they be secured; hence, data security is of central importance in a digital hospital as well as in a PACS environment.

The interfaces shown in Figure 10.1 provide communications between the image acquisition modalities and the HIS/RIS, with the PACS host computer. Through these interfaces, users can also access the PACS host computer. They also provide users to access the PACS computer via the Internet. It is not within the scope of this chapter to describe other PACS components and therefore the interested reader should refer to Seeram [3] for further descriptions of each of the following key characteristics in the functional organization of PACS:

- *Computer networks*: These networks allow information to be transferred and shared among computers, and they consist of both hardware components and the necessary software to enable the hardware to function. Computer networks are classified as local area networks (LANs) or wide area networks (WANs). The basis for this classification is the distance covered by the network. A LAN, for example, connects computers that are separated by short distances such as in a radiology department, a building, or two or more buildings. A WAN, on the other hand, connects computers that are separated by large distances, such as in another province or country. The Internet is a perfect example of a WAN. Other significant system features of computer networks include the bandwidth (data transfer rate); network protocols such as, for example, the Transmission Control Protocol/Internet Protocol (TCP/IP); various servers such as a file server, email server, and a web access server; and network security such as a firewall ("a router, a computer, or even a small network containing routers and computers that is used to connect two networks to provide security" [4]).

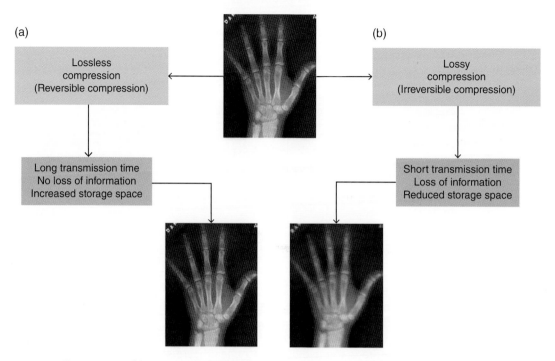

(a)

| Lossless compression (Reversible compression) |

| Lossy compression (Irreversible compression) |

| Long transmission time
No loss of information
Increased storage space |

| Short transmission time
Loss of information
Reduced storage space |

(b)

Figure 10.2   Two types of image compression, namely, lossless compression or reversible compression, where no information is lost in the process, as shown in (a); and lossy compression or irreversible compression, where some information is lost in the process, as shown in (b).

- *Image compression*: Essentially there are two types of image compression, namely, lossless compression or reversible compression, where no information is lost in the process, as shown in Figure 10.2a; and lossy compression or irreversible compression, where some information is lost in the process, as shown in Figure 10.2b. An important concept in image compression is the size of the compressed image, determined by the compression ratio (the ratio between computer storage required to save the original image and that of the compressed data. Thus, a 4 : 1 compression on a $512 \times 8 = 2\,097\,152$ bit image, requires only $524\,288$ bit storage, 25% of the original image storage required. With lossless compression methods yielding ratios of 2 : 1 to 3 : 1 and lossy or irreversible compression having ratios ranging from 10 : 1 to 50 : 1 or more) with lossless compression methods yielding ratios of 2 : 1 to 3 : 1 and lossy or irreversible compression having ratios ranging from 10 : 1 to 50 : 1 or more [5].

- *Image postprocessing:* Apart from image compression, there are other processing functions available in PACS which specifically allow users to change the image brightness and contrast to suit their viewing needs. For example, the postprocessing operation of windowing (gray scale image manipulation) is the most commonly used image manipulation function. The principles of windowing were described in detail in Chapter 8. Other image processing features include edge enhancement and histogram modification. Furthermore, outlining; boundary detection; region of interest (ROI) cleaning; gray scale invert; undo; pixel statistics; zoom and scroll; distance, area, and average gray-level measurements; and annotation. Additionally, image management functions such as delete, auto delete, print, redirect, scrapbook, and mark for teaching, to mention only a few, are also commonplace in PACS.

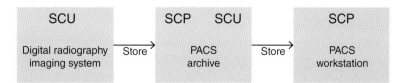

Figure 10.3   An example of one element of DICOM® which identifies a set of essential terminology. DICOM uses the term "role" to indicate that a device can be either a "user" (Service Class User [SCU]) of a service or a "provider" of a service (Service Class Provider [SCP]).

- *The RIS/HIS/PACS broker*: A technical device of the PACS architecture shown in Figure 10.1 is the RIS/PACS broker. This broker facilitates communications between the PACS (image data) with the RIS/HIS (textual data) by linking, for example, the patient's textual data (demographics, etc.) with the same patient's image data in the PACS.
- *The Internet server:* Internet browser technology and microcomputers allow access from within an institution or from outside the institution.
- *Information systems:* Two of these systems shown in Figure 10.1 are the RIS and the HIS. Information systems are computer-based information systems to gather not only medical information about a patient but also all activities related to the hospital's administration, such as billing, accounting, statistics, personnel, budgets, and material management (HIS). The HIS consists of at least two parts: the hospital business and administrative components and the hospital operation component. The RIS on the other hand, could be a stand-alone system, or it may be integrated with a HIS. Examples of functions performed by the RIS in particular are patient registration, examination scheduling, patient tracking, report generation, administration and billing, inventory control, and department statistics.
- *Communication standards:* Two communication standards which are essential features of PACS and information systems are popular and commonplace, HL-7 and the DICOM® standards. As noted earlier, while HL-7 addresses the communication of textual data between the HIS and the RIS and other information systems within the hospital, DICOM deals primarily with the exchange of images in the radiology department and facilitates communication among manufacturer-specific imaging equipment. A description of the elements of DICOM is beyond the scope of this book; however, an example of one such element is illustrated in Figure 10.3 which identifies a set of essential terminology. DICOM uses the term "role" to indicate that a device can be either a "user" (Service Class User [SCU]) of a service or a "provider" of a service (Service Class Provider [SCP]) (Figure 10.3). The interested reader may refer to Seeram [3] for more important and basic elements of DICOM of particular interest to imaging personnel.

IMAGING INFORMATICS

II is defined by the Society for Imaging Informatics in Medicine (SIIM) as ". . .the study and application of processes of information and communications technology for the acquisition, manipulation, analysis, and distribution of image data" [6]. Medical imaging plays a significant role in the healthcare enterprise performing several digital functions (listed in the definition) that require the use of IT, a technology that is rooted in the use of computer technology coupled with communications technology. IT is now a major component of digital medical imaging, including PACS and associated technologies. PACS is without a doubt a part of II.

Through the years from the inception and subsequent growth of PACS to the present, there have been several areas that have received increasing attention in the literature. These areas include enterprise imaging, Big Data, cloud computing, artificial intelligence, and its subsets machine learning (ML) and deep learning (DL).

This section provides a basic overview of these emerging areas of informatics. For a more detailed description of these topics, the student may refer to Seeram [3] and others [7–11]. Each of these will now be examined "at a glance" in order to motivate students and instructors alike to prepare for the further study of II.

Enterprise imaging

The Healthcare Information and Management Systems Society (HIMSS) and SIIM have defined enterprise imaging as "a set of strategies, initiatives and workflows implemented across a healthcare enterprise to consistently and optimally capture, index, manage, store, distribute, view, exchange, and analyze all clinical imaging and multimedia content to enhance the electronic health record" [7].

Cloud computing

Mell and Grence [8] have defined cloud computing as "the access of computing resources through the Internet for purposes of data storage, aggregation, synthesis, and retrieval, together with the capacity to act on the data with computational algorithms and software packages." Additionally, the sharing and data storage have provided the motivation for the development of what has been popularly referred to as "cloud-based PACS" or simply "Cloud PACS." Papadimitroulas et al. [11] describe Cloud PACS as "a PACS system that is located in the cloud and is accessible to both users and administrators though Internet-based user interfaces. Cloud PACS offer the promise of both location and device independence. That is, a Cloud PACS can be accessed by the user from any location, with the assumption that it has sufficient network connectivity and an appropriate connected device that has sufficient display characteristics."

Big Data

Kasandra et al. [9] have described Big Data in detail in their article "Big data and the future of radiology informatics" published in Academic Radiology. They point out that "Big Data refers to extremely complex data sets characterized by the four Vs: Volume, which refers to the sheer number of data elements within these extremely large data sets; Variety, which describes the aggregation of data from multiple sources; Velocity, which refers to the high speed at which data is generated; and Veracity, which describes the inherent uncertainty in some data elements" (Figure 10.4).

Artificial intelligence

Artificial intelligence (AI) belongs to the domain of computer science. The overall goal of AI is "to mimic human cognitive functions" [12]. Two subsets of AI include ML and DL as illustrated in Figure 10.5, which also shows that DL is a subset of ML. Chartrand et al. [13] also provide another definition of AI. They state that AI is "devoted to creating systems to perform tasks that ordinarily require human intelligence."

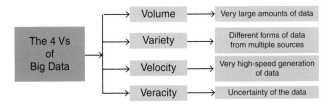

Figure 10.4   The four Vs used to characterize Big Data. See text for further explanation.

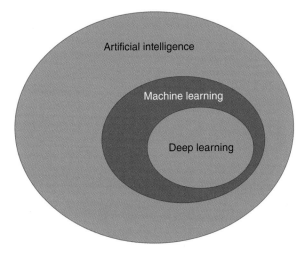

Figure 10.5   Two subsets of AI include machine learning (ML) and deep learning (DL). See text for further description.

Machine learning

Murphy [14] defines ML as "a set of methods that automatically detect patterns in data, and then utilize the uncovered patterns to predict future data or enable decision making under uncertain conditions." Additionally, Erickson et al. [10] point out that in ML, "algorithms are trained to perform tasks by learning patterns from data rather than by explicit programming."

Deep learning

The algorithms used in DL are "characterized by the use of neural networks with many layers" [13], and are "a special type of artificial neural network (ANN) that resembles the multilayered human cognition system" [15].

APPLICATIONS OF AI IN MEDICAL IMAGING

The applications of AI in general range from language understanding, learning, and adaptive systems; problem-solving; perception; modeling; robotics; and games such as chess [16].

The use of AI in healthcare has been examined by Jiang et al. [12], and they list application areas such as medical imaging, genetics, electrodiagnosis, monitoring, physiologic, disability evaluation, mass screening, cancer detection and diagnosis, neurology, and cardiology, for example. In medical imaging, AI is used in enhancing diagnosis and more specifically, in areas such as the detection of the COVID-19 virus [17], and in CT image reconstruction [18, 19].

AI in CT image reconstruction

AI is now being used in CT image reconstruction. In a recent tutorial review paper, Seeram [18] outlines the basics of image reconstruction and focused on the use of AI in CT image reconstruction. Furthermore, a recent systematic review by Lee and Seeram [19] showed that the use of AI is believed to be the next-generation image reconstruction option as current FDA-approved technologies such as General Electric Healthcare's TrueFidelity™ Deep Learning Iterative Reconstruction engine and Canon Medical System's Advanced intelligence Clear-IQ Engine (AiCE) Deep Learning Reconstruction system. These AI-based image reconstruction algorithms have already demonstrated favorable benefits such as dose reduction and improved image quality compared to iterative reconstruction algorithms.

Ethics of AI in radiology

The ethics of AI in radiology have been explored by the European and North America Multi-Society Statement of the American College of Radiology (ACR), the European Society of Radiology, the Radiological Society of North America (RSNA), the SIIM, the European Society of Medical Imaging Informatics, the Canadian Association of Radiologists (CAR), and the American Association of Physicists in Medicine (AAPM). Their summary statement is as follows: "This statement highlights our consensus that ethical use of AI in radiology should promote well-being, minimize harm, and ensure that the benefits and harms are distributed among stakeholders in a just manner. We believe AI should respect human rights and freedoms, including dignity and privacy. It should be designed for maximum transparency and dependability. Ultimate responsibility and accountability for AI remains with its human designers and operators for the foreseeable future. The radiology community should start now to develop codes of ethics and practice for AI that promote any use that helps patients and the common good and should block use of radiology data and algorithms for financial gain without those two attributes" [20].

References

1. Kulikowski, C.A. (1997). Medical imaging informatics: challenges of definition and integration. *J. Am. Med. Inf. Assoc.* 4 (3): 252–253.
2. Samei, E., Seibert, J.A., Andriole, K. et al. (2004). General guidelines for purchasing and acceptance testing of PACS equipment. *Radiographics* 24: 313–334.
3. Seeram, E. (2019). *Digital Radiography: Physical Principles and Quality Control.* Springer Nature Singapore Pte Ltd.
4. Society of Imaging in Medicine (SIIM) (2017). *Innovating Imaging Informatics: Strategic Plan 2017–2020*, 2–13. SIIM.
5. Huang, H.K. (2004). *PACS and Imaging Informatics.* Hoboken, NJ: Wiley.
6. Society for Imaging Informatics in Medicine (2020). What is imaging informatics? https://siim.org (accessed July 2020).
7. Roth, C., Lannum, L., and Persons, K. (2016). A foundation for enterprise imaging: HIMSS-SIIM collaborative white paper. *J. Digit. Imag.* 29: 530–538.

8. Mell, P. and Grence, T. (2011). *The NIST Definition of Cloud Computing*, 800–145. Gaithersburg, MD: U.S. Deptartment of Commerce, National Institute of Standards and Technology. Special Publication.

9. Kansagra, A.P., Yu, J.-P.J., Chatterjee, A.R. et al. (2016). Big data and the future of radiology informatics. *Acad. Radiol.* 23: 30–42.

10. Erickson, B.J., Korfiatis, P., Akkus, Z., and Kline, T.L. (2017). Machine learning. *Radiographics* 37: 505–515.

11. Papadimitroulas, P., Alexakos, C., Nagy, P.G. et al. (2013). Cloud computing in medical imaging. *Med. Phys.* 40 (7): 070901-1–070901-10.

12. Jiang, F., Jiang, Y., Zhi, H. et al. (2017). Artificial intelligence in healthcare: past, present and future. *Stroke Vasc. Neurol.* 2 (4): 230–243.

13. Chartrand, G., Cheng, P.M., Vorontsov, E. et al. (2017). Deep learning: a primer for radiologists. *Radiographics* 37: 2113–2213.

14. Murphy, K.P. (2012). *Machine Learning: A Probabilistic Perspective*, 1e, 25. Cambridge: The MIT Press.

15. Lee, J.-G., Jun, S., Cho, Y.-W. et al. (2017). Deep learning in medical imaging: general overview. *Kor. J. Radiol.* 18 (4): 570–584.

16. Flasinski, M. (2017). *Introduction to Artificial Intelligence*. Cham: Springer International Publishing.

17. Gupta, S. (2020). Artificial intelligence in the era of COVID-19. *Appl. Radiol.* 49 (4): 36–37.

18. Seeram, E. (2020). Computed tomography image reconstruction. *Radiol. Technol.* 92 (2): 155–169.

19. Lee, T. and Seeram, E. (2020). The use of artificial intelligence in computed tomography image reconstruction: a systematic review. *Radiol. Open J.* 5 (1): 1–9.

20. Geis, J.R., Brady, A.P., Wu, C.C. et al. (2019). Ethics of artificial intelligence in radiology: summary of the joint European and north American multisociety statement. *Radiology* 23: 1–5. https://doi.org/10.1148/radiol.2019191586.

SECTION 6
Radiation Protection

11

Basic concepts of radiobiology

"Imaging with gamma and x-rays has saved countless lives over the past century, but medical radiation is a double-edged sword" [1].

The double-edged sword of medical radiation refers to the benefits of imaging vs the risks associated with patients' exposure to ionizing radiation. Weighing the value of diagnostic medical imaging against potential cumulative radiation risk often is referred to as the *risk–benefit ratio*. The benefits of medical imaging are well known based on the work of several investigators [2].

A Comprehensive Guide to Radiographic Sciences and Technology, First Edition. Euclid Seeram.
© 2021 John Wiley & Sons Ltd. Published 2021 by John Wiley & Sons Ltd.

The study of radiobiology involves an extensive list of topics such as, for example, Human Biology, Radiobiological Principles, Molecular and Cellular Radiobiology, and Deterministic and Stochastic Effects [1, 3, 4]. It is not within the scope of this chapter to address details of this wide range of major subject matter. This requires a dedicated course on radiobiology, which is a component of any radiological technology/medical imaging curriculum. The student must therefore refer to the required physics and radiobiology textbooks prescribed by educational programs, for a more detailed description of the topics identified above.

The principal purpose of this chapter therefore is to highlight the essential concepts and principles of radiobiology that serve to support clinical practice and provide a rationale for the optimization of radiation protection of patients, personnel, and members of the public.

WHAT IS RADIOBIOLOGY?

Dr. Elizabeth Travis, Associate Vice President for Women and Minority Faculty Inclusion and Mattie Allen Fair Professor in Cancer Research at the University of Texas, M.D. Anderson Cancer Center, defines *Radiobiology* (also referred to as *Radiation Biology*) as the effects of radiation on biological systems [3]. The sequence of events in which radiation damage in cells occurs and leads to biological effects is illustrated in Figure 11.1. There are at least four important points that are noteworthy: first, there is *damage* to DNA, secondly, *repair* mechanisms follow, and thirdly, damage appears as *cell death/apoptosis* leading to deterministic effects. Finally, repair leads to cell transformations which appear as stochastic effects. *Apoptosis* is cell death caused by a series of molecular changes. A more elaborate scheme leading to biological damage is illustrated in Figure 11.2, and shows those effects which occur days/months (early effects or deterministic effects [non-stochastic effects])and late effects (stochastic effects) which occur years after the exposure.

These effects have been classified into two classes, namely, stochastic effects and deterministic effects. *Stochastic effects* are those effects for which the probability of occurrence depends on the dose and increases as the dose increases linearly, and for which there is no threshold dose (linear non-threshold [LNT] model). Any dose, no matter how small, carries some degree of the risk of injury to the biological system. *Deterministic effects* on the other hand are those effects for which the severity of the effect increases nonlinearly with increasing dose and which there is a threshold dose. This means that there is a given dose, the *threshold dose* (D_T) below which no response is observed. At D_T, a response is observed and it increases as the dose increases. It is important to note that radiation protection standards are based on the LNT model. Dose–response models will be reviewed briefly in this chapter.

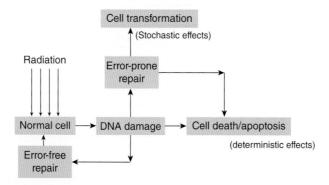

Figure 11.1   The sequence of events in which radiation damage in cells occurs and leads to biological effects. *Source*: Wolbarst et al. [1]. © 2013, John Wiley & Sons.

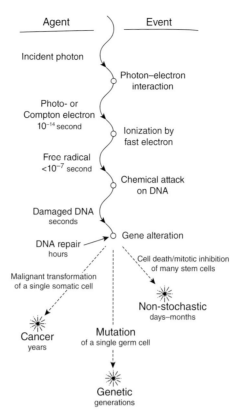

Figure 11.2   A more elaborate scheme leading to biological damage that shows those effects which occur days/months (early effects or deterministic effects [non-stochastic effects]) and late effects (stochastic effects) which occur years after the exposure. *Source*: Wolbarst [5]. Copyright by Dr. Anthony Wolbarst. © 2005, Medical Physics Pub.

BASIC CONCEPTS OF RADIOBIOLOGY

A few examples of essential concepts reviewed briefly in this section include generalizations about radiation effects on living organisms, relevant physical processes, radiosensitivity, dose–response models, radiation effects on target molecule and target theory, direct and indirect effects, DNA and chromosome damage.

Generalizations about radiation effects on living organisms

Travis [3] identifies several generalizations about radiation effects on living organisms to keep in mind. These include:

- The interaction of radiation in cells is a probability function or a matter of chance, that is, an interaction may or may not occur. Furthermore, the occurrence of an interaction does not necessarily mean that damage will result. In fact, damage is frequently repaired.
- The initial deposition of energy occurs very rapidly, within 10^{-18} seconds.
- Radiation deposits energy in a cell in a random fashion.

- Radiation produces no unique changes in cells, tissues, or organs. The changes induced by radiation are indistinguishable from damage produced by other types of trauma.
- The biological changes in cells, tissues, and organs, do not appear immediately. They occur only after a period of time (latent period), ranging from hours (e.g. after accidental exposures to the total body resulting in failure of organ systems and death) to as long as years (e.g. in the case of radiation-induced cancer) or even generations (such as is the case if the damage occurs in a germ cell leading to hereditable changes). The length of the latency period depends on factors related to the radiation, e.g. the dose given, as well as to biological characteristics of the cells irradiated, e.g. how often they divide.

Relevant physical processes

One of the major events leading to biological injury (stochastic and deterministic effects) stems from ionization and excitation, including associated processes of linear energy transfer (LET) and relative biological effectiveness (RBE). The following brief points are noteworthy:

- *Ionization* is the removal of an electron from the atom and this results in the production of *ion pairs*, the ejected electron, and the positively charged atom that remains. Outer shell electrons are easily removed from atoms because they are loosely bound to the nucleus.
- *Excitation* is a physical process in which electrons are raised into other orbital levels due to the absorption of energy from the radiation. Electrons are not removed from the atom. The mechanism of excitation is not fully understood.
- *LET.* This is a physical process which relates to the efficiency of the radiation to cause ionization and excitation. LET measures the rate at which energy is transferred from the radiation to the biological system. LET is measured in kilo-electron volts per micrometer (keV/μm) of length of soft tissue, and as LET increases, biologic damage increases. The LET for diagnostic x-rays is about 3.0 keV/μm. For alpha particles (very damaging radiation), it is 300 keV/μm [4]. As seen in Figure 11.3, *high-LET* radiation (Figure 11.3b) produces more ionizations and free radicals along the path length in tissue, compared to low-LET radiation (Figure 11.3a).
- *RBE.* RBE describes the effectiveness with which different types of radiation can cause biologic damage. The definition of RBE states that it is the ratio of a standard (200–250 kV x-rays) radiation dose required to produce a given bioeffect to the test radiation dose required to produce the same effect. The RBE for diagnostic x-rays is 1. As LET increases, RBE increases, since high LET radiation produces greater ionization, compared with low LET radiation.
- *Radiolysis of water.* Radiolysis of water refers to the breakdown of water by radiation leading to a set of chemical reactions. This is an important point since the body contains about 70–85% water [6]. This interaction results in the ionization of water forming ion pairs and free radicals. Free radicals are highly unstable chemical species and can react to form other chemical species that are harmful to cells. Radiolysis of water was described as early as 1987 by Holahan [6] and summarized by Seeram [7] as follows:
  - $H_2O + radiation \rightarrow H_2O^+ + e^-$.
  - $e^- + H_2O \rightarrow H_2O^-$.
    - Two ions (H_2O^+ and H_2O^-) are the by-products of the initial interaction.
    - Each of these two ions is unstable and exists for only a short time. Each will dissociate as follows:
      - $H_2O^+ \rightarrow H^+ + OH^{\cdot}$.
      - $H_2O^- \rightarrow H^{\cdot} + OH^-$.

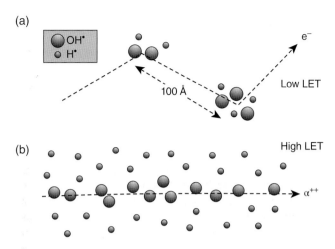

Figure 11.3 High-LET radiation (b) produces more ionizations and free radicals along the path length in tissue, compared to low-LET radiation (a). *Source*: From Wolbarst et al. [1]. © 2013, John Wiley & Sons.

- Now, there are two ions: a hydrogen ion (H⁺) and a hydroxyl ion (OH⁻); and two free radicals: a hydroxyl free radical (OH˙) and a hydrogen free radical (H˙).
- A free radical symbolized by a dot (.), as shown in the above reactions, is an atom or a molecule with an unpaired electron in the outermost orbit.
- Two ions, H⁺ and OH⁻, can recombine as follows:
  - $H^+ + OH^+ \rightarrow H_2O$.
- Free radicals can also recombine as follows:
  - $H˙ + OH˙ \rightarrow H_2O$.
- In the last two cases, water is formed and there is no damage to the cell. However, free radicals can react as follows to form other molecules that are toxic to the cell:
  - $OH˙ + OH˙ \rightarrow H_2O_2$
  - $H˙ + O_2 \rightarrow HO_2˙$
- H_2O_2 is hydrogen peroxide, which is toxic to the cell.
- $HO_2˙$ is hydroperoxyl free radical, which is highly reactive and can be combined with biologic macromolecules to produce more and more free radicals.

Radiosensitivity

Recall the expression for effective dose (E) which states $E = \Sigma W_T H_T$ where W_T relates to the sensitivity of tissues to radiation exposure. This sensitivity is referred to as radiosensitivity. In 1906, Bergonie and Tribondeau, two French scientists, performed experiments to demonstrate this radiosensitivity of various tissues. Their results generated the *Law of Bergonie and Tribondeau*, which states that the radiosensitivity of cells is directly proportional to their level of reproductive activity (proliferation) and inversely proportional to their level of differentiation [6]. This law provides guiding principles for the following as summarized by Seeram [7]:

- Immature cells (stem cells) are more radiosensitive than mature cells (end cells).
- Radiosensitivity is directly proportional to the proliferation rate for cells and the growth rate for tissues. As both rates increase, radiosensitivity increases.
- Young tissues and organs are more radiosensitive than older tissues and organs.

As noted by Bushong [4], this law "serves to remind us that the fetus is considerably more sensitive to radiation exposure than the child or the mature adult."

Radiosensitivity also varies with the phases of the *cell cycle* [6] as follows:

- The most radiosensitive phase is mitosis (M), which includes prophase, metaphase, anaphase, and telophase.
- G_2-phase (post-DNA synthesis) is also extremely sensitive.
- The most radioresistant phase is the S-phase (DNA-synthesis phase). Certain cell types, tissues, and organs are more radiosensitive than are others. For example:
- Spermatogonia, lymphocytes, oocytes erythroblast, hematopoietic stem cells, and the small intestine crypt cells of the gastrointestinal tract have *high radiosensitivity*.
- Hair follicles, colon, stomach, skin, kidney, for example, have *moderate radiosensitivity*.
- Central nervous system (CNS) (neurons), muscle cells, and brain cells have *low radiosensitivity*.

Dose–response models

Several studies [6] have identified dose–risk models or dose–response relationships. These models show what happens to the risk of radiation injury as the dose increases. An important point to note in discussing these models stems from the Radiation Effects Research Foundation (RERF) data, and in this regard, Hendee and O'Connor [8] state that the RERF data "provide statistically significant evidence of increased cancers in Japanese survivors who received doses of 100 mSv and higher, with cancer incidence appearing to increase linearly with dose. At less than 100 mSv, an increase in radiation-induced cancers if any is too small to be distinguishable from cancer incidence due to all causes. Consequently, a model must be deployed to extrapolate from radiation-induced cancers at doses greater than 100 mSv to a hypothetical and much smaller number of cancers induced by doses of a few millisieverts delivered during medical imaging" [8].

The above fact resulted in several dose–response models that extrapolated from high doses to low doses used in medical imaging being proposed. These models have been placed into two categories, namely, the *linear dose–response model without a threshold* (LNT model) and the *nonlinear dose–response model with a threshold*. These models are illustrated in Figure 11.4. The *LNT model* implies that no amount of dose is considered safe, and that any dose, no matter how small, carries some degree of risk. The relationship shows that as the dose increases, the biologic response increases proportionately.

The latter model proposes that no bioeffect is observed below a certain level of dose defined as the threshold dose, and that a biologic response occurs only when the threshold dose is reached, and that the response increases as the dose is increased [4].

The next obvious question in the medical imaging community is which model is best suited to radiation protection of patients. In this regard, our experts [8] state that "the model most widely used is the LNT model. This model is not choses because there is solid biologic or epidemiologic data supporting its use. Rather, it is used because of its simplicity and because it is a conservative approach (that is, if it is not correct, then it probably overestimates the risk of cancer induction at low dose). For the purpose of establishing radiation protection standards for occupationally exposed individuals and members of the public, a conservative model which overestimates the risk is preferred over a model that underestimates risk" [8].

This section would not be complete without some mention of the current debate concerns among the scientific and imaging communities. In the regard, a literature review of this topic was done by Tran and Seeram [9] examining this situation. In summary, the review showed that there are concerns about the data obtained from epidemiological studies as well as the consequence effects of the LNT model on the public. In response, alternative dose–response models that

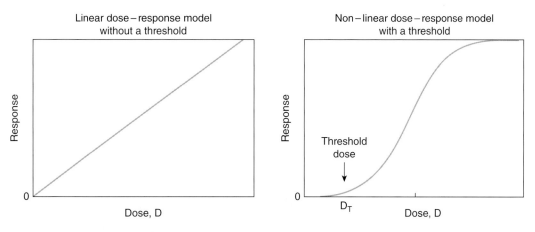

Figure 11.4 Two categories of dose–response models: the linear dose–response model without a threshold (LNT model) and the nonlinear dose–response model with a threshold. See text for further explanation.

contradict the accepted LNT model especially at low doses have been suggested. Furthermore, the review showed that more research is needed on the effects of low doses on specific organs and tissue to further quantify risk estimates.

Finally, on this issue, the Health Physics Society in a special issue of the *Journal of Health Physics* (The *Radiation Safety* Journal) [10] presented the summaries of several papers addressing "The Applicability of Radiation-Response Models to Low-Dose Protection Standards." One paper, in particular, entitled "ICRP Views on Radiation Risk at Low Doses Through the Lens of Fukushima" presented by Christopher Clement [10], Scientific Secretary of the International Commission on Radiological Protection (ICRP), noted several important points including the following on the LNT model (and within the context of this section of this chapter) are:

- "LNT as 'a prudent basis for radiological protection' makes summation of doses possible and drives optimization of protection. At high doses, risk is higher, and at low doses, risk is lower. Action should be commensurate with dose/risk. At low doses, action, if any, should be modest" [10].
- "LNT is not meant to be accurate. It is meant to be a reasonable model for protection" [10].

Radiation interactions in tissue: target theory, direct and indirect action

There is strong evidence that biological effects of radiation exposure including cell death, mutagenesis, and carcinogenesis are due to damage primarily to one molecule, DNA. DNA therefore has been called the *critical target*. Radiation may deposit energy directly within the critical target, or conversely, may interact with other molecules in the cell; one of the most important is water. There are three considerations that are important in this regard:

The target theory
This theory states that inactivation of the critical target molecule (DNA) after irradiation will cause the cell to die. The site of this interaction determines whether the initial interaction is direct or indirect.

Direct action

This action occurs when radiation is absorbed by the molecule known to be critical to maintaining the life of the cell (e.g. DNA), as illustrated in Figure 11.5, thus initiating a series of events, leading to changes that may be lethal to the cell.

Indirect action

This action occurs when the radiation interacts with other molecules in the cell, most notably, water, as illustrated in Figure 11.5. Since the cell consists of about 70–85% water [6], the majority of interactions occur via indirect action.

Although there are a number of free radicals that may be produced as a result of indirect action, the oxidizing agent OH is considered the most damaging. It is estimated to account for about two-thirds all of x-ray damage to DNA in mammalian cells. Although both direct and indirect actions initiate a series of molecular, biochemical, and biological events that lead to the overt expression of damage over a course of months to years later, these interactions remain poorly understood [3].

DNA and chromosome damage

An overview of the particular damage to DNA and chromosomes are briefly outlined in the next section.

DNA damage

As stated earlier, DNA is a critical target. Experiments show that lower doses of radiation are needed to induce cell death when only the nucleus is irradiated than when the cytoplasm is irradiated. DNA is made up of two strands forming a double helix composed of sugar base pairs of adenine, guanine, cytosine, and thiamine. Irradiation of DNA can result in the following events:

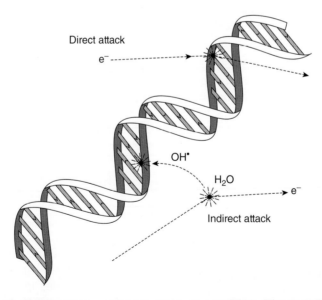

Direct attack

e^-

$OH^\bullet$

H_2O

e^-

Indirect attack

Figure 11.5   Direct and indirect action on the target molecule DNA. Direct action occurs when radiation is absorbed by the DNA, thus initiating a series of events, leading to changes that may be lethal to the cell. Indirect action occurs when the radiation interacts with other molecules in the cell, most notably, water. Since the cell consists of about 70–85% water, the majority of interactions occur via indirect action. *Source*: From Wolbarst et al. [1]. © 2013, John Wiley & Sons.

- Single-strand breaks or double-strand breaks.
- Both breaks can be repaired.
- Single-strand breaks are less damaging than double-strand breaks, which can lead to cell death.
- Loss or change of base that leads to genetic mutations.
- Interstrand crosslink resulting in a separation of bases.

The previously mentioned lesions produced in DNA by irradiation result in cell death, malignant disease, and genetic effects. For a more detailed description of the interaction of x-rays with DNA, the interested reader should refer to Seeram and Brennan [6].

Chromosome damage

Chromosomes contain DNA, and damage to DNA leads to chromosome damage. Chromosome damage is also referred to as chromosome aberrations (or breaks) [6, 7]. These aberrations as summarized by Seeram [7] are:

- *Single-hit aberrations*, which can occur via the direct or indirect effect. The hit, which is an interaction of radiation with the chromosome, will cause a noticeable derangement of the chromosome. Examples of single-hit aberrations include chromatid breaks and chromosome deletions.
- *Multi-hit aberrations*, which result in dicentrics, ring chromosomes, multicentrics, and reciprocal translocations.

Experiments have demonstrated that these chromosome aberrations lead to malignancies such as Burkitt's lymphoma, acute promyelocytic leukemia, and ovarian cancer. Chromosome deletions, specifically, lead to small cell lung cancer, neuroblastoma, retinoblastoma, and Wilms' tumor [3].

EFFECTS OF RADIATION EXPOSURE TO THE TOTAL BODY

Experiments on whole-body irradiation have been conducted on animals. Furthermore, humans have experienced whole-body irradiation, and the effects, known as acute effects, are well documented. For example, data on humans have boon obtained from individuals exposed at Hiroshima and Nagasaki, the Marshall Islanders exposed to fallout radiation, nuclear accident victims such as Chernobyl, for example, and patients undergoing radiation therapy. In 2011, there was a nuclear reactor meltdown at Fukushima, Japan, and fortunately, "no acute lethality was observed" [4]. The major effect of high acute exposures to the whole body is lethality occurring within days to weeks after the exposure. Lethality is described by the term lethal dose. For example, the dose required to kill 50% of the human population in 60 days is termed the *lethal dose 50/60* ($LD_{50/60}$). For humans, the $LD_{50/60}$ is 3.5 Gy (350 rad) [4].

The time of death is dependent on the dose given and is preceded by a specific set of signs and symptoms that is directly related to damage and cell death in a particular system. This condition is described by the term *total body syndrome* or *radiation syndrome*. Three distinct syndromes have been defined after whole-body irradiation resulting from damage to three specific organ systems, namely, the *central nervous system syndrome*, the *gastrointestinal syndrome*, and the *hematopoietic or bone marrow syndrome*. These syndromes have been plotted as a graph which shows the relationship between the dose and the survival time for each of these three syndromes. The time of death depends on the magnitude of the dose received. The higher the dose, the earlier death occurs. The dose and the organ systems affected have been described in detail by Travis [3], Bushong [4], and Bushberg et al. [11], and are summarized by Seeram [7] in the following subsections:

Hematopoietic of bone marrow syndrome

This syndrome occurs after an acute whole-body exposure of 2–10 Gy. The dose affects the stem cells in the bone marrow and other blood-forming organs.

Gastrointestinal syndrome

This syndrome occurs after an acute whole-body exposure of doses between 10 and 100 Gy. Damage to the crypt cells of the small intestines will cause death, which occurs much faster than that caused by the bone marrow syndrome.

Central nervous system (CNS) syndrome

The CNS syndrome requires doses in excess of 100 Gy. Death results because blood vessels in the brain are damaged, leading to edema that causes an increase in skull pressure.

DETERMINISTIC EFFECTS

Earlier in this chapter, the class of biological effects following radiation exposure was defined as those effects for which the severity (rather than the probability) of the effect increases with increases dose, and there is a threshold dose (D_T). It was also stated that these effects follow a nonlinear dose–response relationship. These effects, which appear at *high doses* (beyond the doses used in diagnostic x-ray imaging) are referred to as *deterministic effects*, and have been observed in animals as well as humans, and appear within a few days to months after the exposure. Because of this, these effects have also been called *early effects*. Examples of these effects on humans and the approximate D_T are as follows [4]:

- *Death* as a result of whole-body exposure. Approximate D_T is 2 Gy (200 rad).
- *Skin erythema (reddening)*. Small field exposure. Approximate D_T is 2 Gy (200 rad).
- *Epilation*. Small field exposure. Approximate D_T is 3 Gy (300 rad).
- *Hematologic depression*. Whole-body exposure. Approximate D_T is 250 mGy (25 rad).
- *Gonadal dysfunction*. Local tissue exposure. Approximate D_T is 100 mGy (10 rad).
- *Chromosome aberration*. Whole-body exposure. Approximate D_T is 50 mGy (5 rad).

The following points are noteworthy regarding the radiation effects on the gonads and the hemopoietic system as described in detail by Travis [3], Bushong [4], Bushberg et al. [11], and summarized by Seeram [7] as follows:

- The principal effect of high doses of radiation on the gonads (*ovaries and testes*) is atrophy (reduction in size). In women, the *oocyte* is highly radiosensitive. Radiation exposure of the ovaries can delay or suppress menstruation, as well as cause temporary or permanent sterility. A dose of 2 Gy will cause *temporary sterility*; 5 Gy will cause *permanent sterility*.
- In men, the *spermatogonia* are most radiosensitive compared with spermatocytes and spermatids. A dose of 100 mGy decreases the spermatozoa count. A dose of 2 Gy produces *temporary sterility*; 5 Gy will produce *permanent sterility*. Spermatogonia are also considered to be among the most radiosensitive of body cells (as well as lymphocytes).

- The *blood system* or *hemopoietic system* is made up of the *bone marrow, lymphoid tissue, and circulating blood*. The main effect of radiation on this system is to reduce the number of blood cells in the peripheral circulation. Among the blood cells, *lymphocytes* are the most radiosensitive.

STOCHASTIC EFFECTS

Another class of biological effects following radiation exposure is stochastic effects, defined as those effects for which the probability of occurrence depends on the dose and increases linearly as the dose increases, and for which there is no threshold dose. Stochastic effects follow the LNT dose–response model, described above. The general conclusion drawn from this relationship is that any dose, no matter how small, carries some degree of the risk of injury to the biological system. These effects occur years after the exposure and for this reason they are also referred to as *stochastic effects* or *late effects*. Furthermore, the doses received in diagnostic imaging are low and have a low LET. Additionally, the doses to patients are low and "are delivered intermittently over long periods" [4].

Several authors [3, 4, 11], for example, have described these effects in detail and the interested reader must refer to these references for a more in-depth discussion of the various mechanisms involved. As noted by Bushong [4], "the principal stochastic effects of low-dose radiation over long periods consist of radiation-induced malignancy and genetic effects. Life-span shortening and effects on local tissues have also been reported as stochastic effects, but these are not considered significant."

Tissue effects

These effects are non-malignancies that can appear in the skin, eyes, and chromosomes. "The *skin* develops a weathered, callused, and discolored appearance" [4]. Damage has been observed in the *chromosomes* of circulatory lymphocytes. *Cataracts* (opacification of the lens fibers in the eyes) have also been observed in the eye as a late effect of radiation. It is important to note that these effects are not significant in diagnostic radiology, except for skin damage from patients who may have lengthy interventional angiographic procedures.

Life-span shortening

There is no need for radiologists and technologists working in diagnostic radiology to be concerned about life-span effects. Bushong [4] notes that "at worst, humans can expect a reduced life span of approximately 10 days for every ao mGy." Additionally, the expected days of life lost being male rather than female, heart disease, being unmarried, smoking one pack of cigarettes per day, cancer, motor vehicle accidents, and radiation worker are 2800, 2100, 2000, 1000, 980, 200, and 12 days, respectively [4].

Radiation-induced cancers

The first case of radiation-induced cancer was reported 6 years after Roentgen's discovery; within 15 years, 100 cases of skin cancer were reported in occupationally exposed persons.

Since these early reports, a large body of data has been collected, indicating that radiation does cause cancer. The most compelling data regarding the carcinogenic effect of radiation in humans are derived from the following [3]:

* Increased incidence of many types of cancer, including leukemia, and many types of solid tumors, in survivors of the atomic bombings of Hiroshima and Nagasaki.
* Increased incidence of leukemia in irradiated patients with ankylosing spondylitis.
* Increased incidence of leukemia in radiologists.
* Increased incidence of thyroid cancer in children irradiated for ringworm or for enlarged thymus.

Cancer induction is the most significant stochastic effect of radiation. The evidence stems from radium dial painters, uranium miners, atomic bomb survivors, patients exposed to radiation in fluoroscopy, and for ankylosing spondylitis [3, 4, 11].

Furthermore, cancer induction is associated with tissues and organs that are highly radiosensitive, such as the lymphoid tissue, bone marrow, the breast and gonads, and the gastrointestinal tract. Radiation-induced cancers include leukemia (the incidence of leukemia is dependent on the dose (incidences increase with increased dose). Leukemia may appear two to three years after exposure, lung cancer, breast cancer, thyroid cancer, bone cancer, and liver cancer [3, 4, 6, 11].

Travis [3] notes that the mechanism of radiation-induced cancer can be explained by molecular biology strengthening understanding of the molecular genetics of cancer. There are three mechanisms by which radiation may induce changes leading to cancer: checkpoint genes that control cellular proliferation and differentiation may be disrupted, or cells may be converted from normal to malignant, or by either the activation of oncogenes or loss of suppressor genes. In some cancers, more than one of these mechanisms may be involved [3].

Hereditary effects

Hereditary effects are stochastic or late effects that occur in the offspring of the irradiated individual. Irradiation of germ cells (spermatozoa or ova) can result in chromosomal mutations, and gene mutations. Chromosomal mutations have been associated with a number of diseases and include aberrations or changes in chromosome distribution (e.g. Down's syndrome, in which there is an extra chromosome 23) [3]. "Gene mutations, on the other hand, can be a change in the composition or the sequence of bases, or both on the DNA molecule. It might seem unlikely that small alterations in the DNA can cause significant changes in the individual, but this is not true. Sickle cell anemia, for example, results from the substitution of a single base on the DNA. Thus, radiation can cause profound changes in the genome, which can be passed on to future generations" [3]. Genetic effects of radiation have been studied extensively in animals, the results of which have been extrapolated to humans because the data for humans are limited. As Travis [3] points out:

* Most mutations are harmful.
* Any dose of radiation, no matter how small, can cause genetic changes.
* There is a linear relationship between dose and the number of mutations, thus information after low doses can be extrapolated from high-dose data.
* Man is not more sensitive than mouse and may in fact be less sensitive.
* Mouse data can provide reasonable estimates of the risk of radiation-induced genetic effects in humans.

RADIATION EXPOSURE DURING PREGNANCY

This topic has been described by several authors [3, 4, 6, 11], and it is vital that the interested reader consult these references. For example, Travis [3] has discussed the essential points relating to the effects of radiation on the embryo and fetus, by outlining the classic triad of radiologic, embryologic syndromes, and the fetal development and radiation effects.

The data for the information and knowledge concerning the effects of radiation on the developing fetus and embryo is derived from studies in mice and rats, because these animals have large liters and the gestational times are short. Furthermore, data from humans on the effects of irradiation at various stages of human gestation are also available and these are from 1600 survivors irradiated in utero from Hiroshima and Nagasaki atomic bombings.

The human embryo and fetus are highly sensitive to radiation, thus every effort must be made to protect them from unnecessary radiation exposure. A recent review on "Ionizing Radiation Exposure During Pregnancy: Effects on Postnatal Development and Life" by Sreetharan et al. [12] and published in *Radiation Research* Journal provides the following summary:

> There is a major consensus that the atomic bomb survivors' data shows increased incidence of microcephaly and reductions in Intelligence Quotient (IQ) of A-bomb survivors, whereas, with diagnostic radiography in utero there is no conclusive evidence of increased cancer risk. Due to the relatively limited data (particularly for low-dose exposures) in humans, animal models have emerged as an important tool to study prenatal effects of radiation. These animal models enable researchers to manipulate various experimental parameters and make it possible to analyze a wider variety of end points. In this review, we discuss the major findings from studies using mouse and rat models to examine prenatal ionizing radiation effects in postnatal development of the offspring. In addition, we broadly categorize trends across studies within three major stages of development: pre-implantation, organogenesis and fetal development. Overall, long-term effects of prenatal radiation exposure (including the possible role on the developmental programing of disease) are important factors to consider when assessing radiation risk, since these effects are of relevance even in the low-dose range.

References

1. Wolbarst, A.B., Capasso, P., and Wyant, A.R. (2013). *Medical Imaging: Essentials for Physicians*. Hoboken, NJ: Wiley.
2. Hricak, H., Brenner, D.J., Adelstein, S.J. et al. (2011). Managing radiation use in medical imaging: a multifaceted challenge. *Radiology* 258 (3): 889–905.
3. Travis, E. (1997). Bioeffects of radiation. In: *Radiation Protection* (ed. E. Seeram). Philadelphia, NY: Lippincott.
4. Bushong, S. (2017). *Radiologic Science for Technologists*, 11e. St Louis, MO: Elsevier.
5. Wolbarst, A.B. (2005). *Physics of Radiology*, 2e. Medical Physics Pub Corp.
6. Seeram, E. and Brennan, P. (2017). *Radiation Protection in Diagnostic X-Ray Imaging*. Burlington, MA: Jones and Bartlett Learning.
7. Seeram, E. (2020). *Rad Tech's Guide to Radiation Protection*. Oxford: Wiley.
8. Hendee, W.R. and O'Connor, M.K. (2013). Radiation risks of medical imaging: separating fact from fantasy. *Radiology* 204 (2): 312–320.
9. Tran, L. and Seeram, E. (2017). Current perspectives on the use of the linear non-threshold (LNT) in radiation protection. *Int. J. Radiol. Med. Imag.* 3: 123–128.

10. Clement, C. (2020). ICRP views on radiation risk at low doses through the lens of Fukushima. *Health Phys.* 118 (3): 311–316.

11. Bushberg, J.T., Seibert, J.A., Leidholdt, E.M. Jr., and Boone, J.M. (2011). *The Essential Physics of Medical Imaging*. Philadelphia: Wolters Kluwer/Lippincott Williams & Wilkins.

12. Sreetharan, S., Thorne, C., Tharmalingham, S. et al. (2017). Ionizing radiation exposure during pregnancy: effects on postnatal development and life. *Radiat. Res.* 187: 647–658.

12

Technical dose factors in radiography, fluoroscopy, and CT

A significant factor in radiation protection of the patient in digital radiography, fluoroscopy, and computed tomography (CT) is that of the operator (technologist, radiographer, and radiologist) must have a good understanding of the technical factors affecting the dose delivered to the patient. This skill enables the operator to work within the International Commission on Radiological Protection (ICRP) optimization principle, meaning that the dose to the patient must be as low as reasonably achievable (ALARA) and not compromise image quality.

The purpose of this chapter is to outline the major technical factors that affect dose to the patient during radiography, fluoroscopy, and CT.

DOSE FACTORS IN DIGITAL RADIOGRAPHY

The general radiographic system components affecting the dose to the patient during an examination are illustrated in Figure 12.1. Major components include the x-ray generator, the x-ray tube, x-ray beam filter, the x-ray beam collimator, the x-ray beam area (field-of-view), patient thickness and density, table top, scattered radiation grid, the image receptor (detector), source-to-skin distance (SSD), source-to-image receptor distance (SID), and finally, the operator who has direct control of the x-ray beam quantity, determined by the mAs, and beam quality, determined by the kV, needed for the examination. These are the exposure technique factors.

It is clear in Figure 12.1 that there are several technical factors affecting patient dose in diagnostic radiography, some of which are under the direct control of the operator and others that are not. For example, the type of x-ray generator and x-ray tube characteristics are not under the control of the operator. However, those factors under the direct control of the operator include the exposure technique factors, collimation and field size, beam alignment, SID, SSD, and image receptor selection. The influence of each of the factors on dose will now be described briefly.

The x-ray generator

The x-ray generator was described in Chapter 4. These generators have evolved from low-powered (single-phase generators) to high-powered generators (high-frequency generators). The major goal of this evolution is to improve the efficiency of x-ray production in an effort to

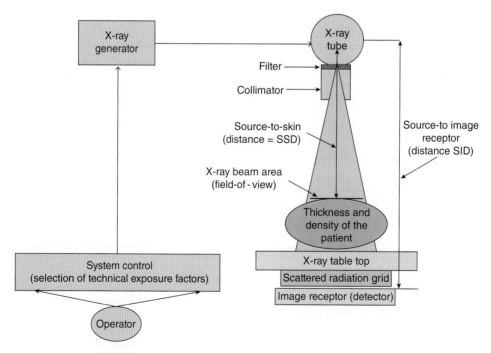

Figure 12.1   The general radiographic system components affecting the dose to the patient during an examination. See text for further details.

reduce the dose delivered to the patient. This efficiency refers to the patient dose and hence the exposure technique factors (kVp and mAs) are related to the type of voltage waveform. State-of-the-art x-ray generators are high-frequency generators, since they are much more efficient at x-ray production than three-phase and single-phase x-ray generators. The high-frequency generator, however, produces greater x-ray intensity. This means that shorter exposure times (hence mAs) are possible. Bushong [1] notes that "The relationship between x-ray quantity and the type of high-voltage generator provides the basis for another rule of thumb used by radiologic technologists. If a radiographic technique calls for 72 kV on single-phase equipment, then on three-phase equipment, approximately 64 kV – a 12% reduction – will produce similar results."

Exposure technique factors

Exposure technique factors refer to the kV, mA, and the time in seconds (s). These three factors (kV, mA, and time) not only determine the quality (kV) and quantity (mA×s = mAs) of the radiation beam needed to image the patient, but they also affect the dose to the patient. The relationships to dose are as follows:

- Dose is directly proportional to the mA. Doubling the mA will double the dose.
- Dose is directly proportional to the time of exposure. Doubling the time will double the dose.
- Dose α [kV_{new}/kV_{old}] [2]. If the mA is held constant, the dose increases by about 50% if the kV is increased from 120 to 140 kV. On the other hand, the dose decreases by about 65% if the kV is reduced from 120 to 80 kV [2].
- Techniques based on high kV require a subsequent reduction in mAs; hence, high kV techniques result in reduced dose to the patient.

X-ray beam filtration

The x-ray beam emerging from the x-ray tube is a heterogeneous beam. This means that the beam consists of low-energy and high-energy photons. Whereas the high-energy photons penetrate the patient to form the image at the image receptor, low-energy photons do not have enough energy to penetrate the patient and they do not therefore play a role in image formation. They are merely absorbed by the tissues, thus increasing the dose to the patient. *Filtration* is a strategy to removing or absorbing these low-energy photons by inserting metal absorbers in the beam. These absorbers are called *filters* (Figure 12.1).

- *Filtration* is required by regulatory radiation protection authorities and must be present to protect the patient. Filtration results in a reduction of the intensity (quantity) and an increase in the effective energy of the beam; that is, the beam becomes harder and therefore more penetrating.
- The *total filtration* (inherent filtration due to x-ray tube design + additional filtration) in diagnostic radiographic imaging is generally 2.5 aluminum (Al); 0.5 mm Al equivalent inherent plus 1.0 mm Al added plus 1.0 mm Al equivalent of the mirror in the collimator [1].
- Copper (Cu) and tin (Sn) as well as rare earth filters such as gadolinium and holmium may also be used as filters, depending on their clinical applications. For example, rare earth filters are commonplace in pediatric imaging.

Collimation and field size

The position of the collimator is shown in Figure 12.1. *Collimation* shapes and limits the x-ray beam to area of interest (the anatomy of interest). This area is also referred to as the field size.

This action therefore is intended to protect the patient from unnecessary radiation. A few important points about collimation are:

- The *surface integral exposure* (total radiation) is directly proportional to the size of the irradiated area (*field size*).
- An approach is automatic collimation in *positive-beam-limitation* (PBL) where the beam is automatically collimated to the size of the image receptor in the Bucky tray. PBL can be overridden by the technologist to ensure that the beam can be collimated to a size smaller than the image receptor size.
- Collimation also decreases not only the bone marrow and gonadal doses but reduces the genetically significant dose by about 65% [1].
- An interesting study by Fauber and Dempsey [3] showed that when the x-ray field size decreased from 14×17 in (35×43 cm) to 8×17 in (20×43 cm), a 27% dose reduction is obtained.
- Beam alignment means that the radiation field from the x-ray tube, and the light field from the collimator must be congruent; that is, they must be in perfect alignment. Improper alignment will result in unnecessary radiation to the patient due to beam overlap. The quality control test for beam alignment tolerance limit states that the misalignment must not exceed 2% of the SID [1].
- In digital radiography, a postprocessing technique known as *electronic collimation* uses digital shutters to electronically collimate the image after the patient has been x-rayed. With respect to this approach, Bomer et al. [4] offer two noteworthy points.
  - "Electronic collimation implies that the original field size should have been smaller and the child has been exposed to unnecessary radiation."
- Furthermore, Bomer et al. [4] conclude that "The ability to electronically collimate an image after acquisition carries the risk of over exposure . . . If the field size has been overestimated, we can use electronic collimation to optimize image quality. However, the original images should always be sent to the PACS (picture archiving and communications systems), as they may contain critically important information and the patient has a right to all information at all times."

The SID and SSD

The SID and the SSD are illustrated in Figure 12.1. For most radiographic examinations, the SID is usually set at 101 cm (40 in.). A short SID increases the photon concentration, thus increasing the surface exposure to the patient. This is graphically shown in Figure 12.2. The following point is noteworthy:

- A study by Joyce et al. [5] showed that by increasing the SID from 100 to 150 cm resulted in a statistically significant reduction in effective dose (ED) between 19.2 and 23% ($p \leq 0.05$) without compromising image quality.

Patient thickness and density

The technologist has no control over the patient thickness and density. These two factors do affect the dose to the patient in that as these factors increase, more dose is required to maintain acceptable image quality.

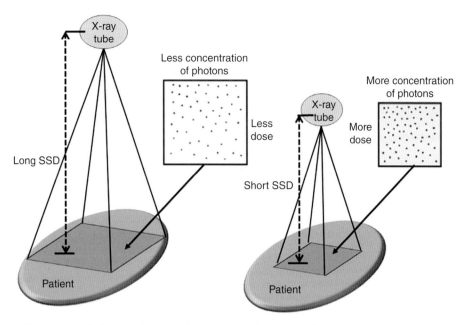

Figure 12.2   The effect of SID on dose to the patient. A short SID increases the photon concentration, thus increasing the surface exposure to the patient.

Scattered radiation grid

The purpose of a scattered radiation grid (anti-scatter grid) is to improve radiographic contrast, by absorbing and preventing the scattered rays from the patient before they fall onto the detector. This goal depends on several design characteristics of the grid, such as the grid ratio, the interspace material, grid frequency, selectivity, and the Bucky factor. For a detailed description of the design characteristics of the anti-scatter, the reader should refer to the textbook by Bushong [1]. These factors affect dose to the patient in the following manner:

- As the grid ratio increases (ratio of the height of the lead strip to the distance between the strips), the dose increases. Furthermore, a moving grid (found in Bucky mechanisms) requires about 15% more radiation than a stationary grid with the same design characteristics [1].
- The *interspace material* of the grid supports the lead strips and provides an equal amount of separation between them. The interspace material is usually aluminum or plastic fiber. While each of these has its advantages, aluminum, with its high atomic number, absorbs more radiation than the plastic fiber, especially when using low kV techniques. This feature will result in an increase in the patient dose by about 20% [1].
- The *grid frequency* is the number of lead strips per cm of the grid. The grid frequency is also referred to as the grid lattice or strip density. Grid frequencies range from 24 to 43 lines per cm, although higher strip densities are available. As the grid frequency increases, the relative patient exposure increases, because there is more lead which absorbs a small proportion of the primary radiation beam.
- *Selectivity* is defined as the ratio of primary radiation transmission to scattered radiation transmission. Selectivity depends on not only the grid ratio but also on the amount of lead used in the construction of the grid. In general, grids with high selectivity will result in higher patient doses, because of an increase in the thickness of the lead strips [1].

- The Bucky factor (B) (or grid factor) is defined as the ratio of the incident total radiation striking the grid (primary plus scatter) to the total radiation transmitted through the grid [6]. B is related to the grid ratio as well as the kV. As the grid ratio and kV increase, B increases. For example, the B for a 12 : 1 grid is 3.5, 4, and 5 at 70, 90, and 120 kV, respectively. As B increases, patient dose increases proportionally [1].

The sensitivity of the image receptor

The *sensitivity* (S) of the image receptor (detector) refers to the speed; that is, the amount of radiation needed to produce acceptable images. A high-speed detector requires less radiation than a low-speed detector. S is inversely proportional to the radiation dose. The higher the sensitivity, the less dose needed to produce images. For digital radiography systems, the term speed does not apply, since the digital detector operates on any *speed class.*

An equivalent or related characteristic is the detective quantum efficiency (DQE), as described in Chapter 8. The digital detector takes an input exposure and converts it into a useful output image. The DQE is a measure of the efficiency with which the detector performs this task. The DQE for a perfect detector is 1 or 100% [6]. This means that there is no loss of information.

DOSE FACTORS IN FLUOROSCOPY

The system components and how they function to perform fluoroscopy were described in Chapter 4 for image intensifier-based fluoroscopy and digital fluoroscopy, the major components of which are shown in Figure 12.3. Since the former systems may still be used in some places, the latter has replaced the former system. In general, fluoroscopy systems are now all digital.

There are two major categories of technical factors affecting dose in fluoroscopy and they include *Fluoroscopic Exposure Factors* and *Fluoroscopic Instrumentation Factors* [8].

Fluoroscopic exposure factors

These factors are the exposure technique factors and refer to the kV, mA, and time in seconds (s) used during a fluoroscopic examination. These factors create the image displayed on the television monitor. The influence of kV and mAs on dose has been described in subsection "Exposure Technique Factors" for radiographic imaging. Important points to note about the use of kV and mA, and the time of exposure are as follows:

- *Fluoroscopic factors* are generally low mA and high kV, with a range of 1–3 mA and 65–120 kV depending on the examination. For example, a single-contrast barium enema requires a range of 110–120 kV while a range of 50–90 kV is acceptable for a double-contrast (air-contrast) barium enema [1].
- *Fluoroscopic mA* used in image intensifier fluoroscopy systems ranges from 1 to 3 mA.
- For *digital fluoroscopy systems*, the mA is measured in hundreds of mA instead of <5 mA [1]. To address the dose increases from the use of hundreds of mA, a technique known as *pulse-progressive fluoroscopy* is used.
- The *fluoroscopic exposure time* can range from minutes to hours depending on the examination. In light of these high exposures, it is important for the operator to limit the "beam on"

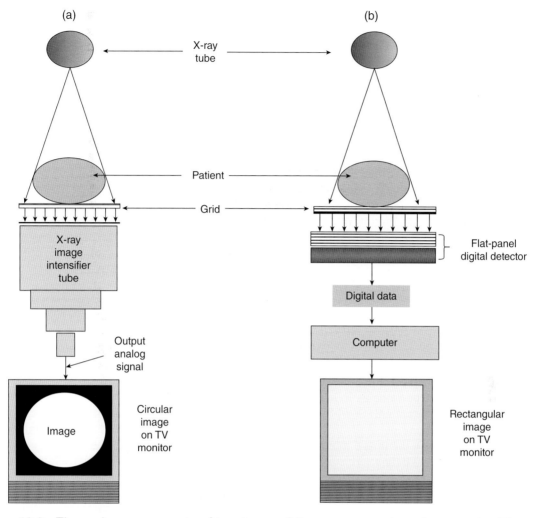

(a)   (b)

X-ray tube

Patient

Grid

X-ray image intensifier tube

Flat-panel digital detector

Digital data

Output analog signal

Computer

Image

Circular image on TV monitor

Rectangular image on TV monitor

Figure 12.3   The major components of two types of fluoroscopy systems in use today. The system is shown in (a), while the newer system is shown in (b). *Source*: Seeram [7]. © 2020, John Wiley & Sons.

time (fluoroscopy time) by *using intermittent fluoroscopy* (short bursts of "beam on" time) rather than continuous fluoroscopy, described in the next section.

- Fluoroscopic systems are equipped with a *cumulative timer* not only to keep track of the "beam-on" time, but also to remind the operator of each three-minute maximum (for modern units) time period of exposures via an audible sound. When this sound occurs, fluoroscopy ceases, until the timer is reset to begin another three minutes of exposure.

Fluoroscopic equipment factors

These factors include the modes of operation, dose level control, automatic exposure rate control (AERC), collimation, anti-scatter grids, filtration, magnification (geometric and electronic), and last image hold (LIH). The following summaries are important to remember:

- There are two methods in which fluoroscopic systems can operate: while older units operate used a *continuous fluoroscopy mode*, digital fluoroscopy systems operate in the *variable frame-rate pulsed fluoroscopy*. The continuous fluoroscopy mode of operation involves the production of a continuous x-ray beam. The pulsed fluoroscopy mode allows for the x-ray generator to produce x-rays in shorts bursts (pulses) rather than continuously. The frames per second (FPS) are typically 30, 15, 7.5, and 3.75 FPS. These variable frame rates allow the operator to select the appropriate frame rate with dose reduction in mind; the higher the FPS, the greater the radiation dose. A frame rate of 7.5 FPS reduces the dose to 25% (7.5/30) [9].

- The overall goal of pulsed fluoroscopy is to reduce the dose to the patient, and this is reflected in a study that showed dose reduction of 64% and a reduction of fluoroscopic time by 76%, compared to continuous fluoroscopy [10].

- AERC is a new term that has replaced the term automatic brightness control (ABC). AERC is a technique designed to maintain the brightness of the imaged displayed on the television screen when the anatomical part thickness changes; that is, when the patient changes from say the AP position to the oblique and subsequently to the lateral positions. Furthermore, when the beam moves from a thick part to a thin part, dose is decreased to the thin part. AERC also plays an important role in maintaining constant signal-to-noise ratio (SNR) in the image, by altering the mA and kV automatically as the thickness of the patient varies in the beam path, thus resulting in dose control.

- Collimation in fluoroscopy is no different than collimation in radiography. The fluoroscopic beam should always be collimated to the anatomy of interest. While this strategy will limit the dose to the patient, it also ensures good image quality, by reducing the amount of scattered radiation reaching the detector.

- The SSD is the same as in radiography and is the distance from the x-ray focal spot to the surface of the patient. Short SSDs will result in more dose to the patient since the concentration of photons per unit area is greatest compared to longer SSDs. The patient dose is reduced when the image intensifier tube is close to the patient and the x-ray tube is farther away from the patient. This arrangement represents the best beam geometry to use in fluoroscopy. A poor geometry is one in which the x-ray tube is too close to the patient thus resulting in a greater dose compared to a situation where the detector (digital detector or image intensifier) is close to the patient using the same SSD. The final geometry represents a situation where digital detector (or the image intensifier tube) is too far away from the patient, thus increasing the dose compared to a situation where the detector is close to the patient during imaging.

- The *patient size* affects the dose during the examination. Thicker patients will require more exposure (kV and mA) to penetrate the body part to produce optimal image brightness, detail, and contrast, compared with thinner patients.

- *Image magnification* in fluoroscopy is yet another equipment-related factor that affects the dose to the patient. The basic elements of magnification were described in Chapter 6. Magnification can be accomplished by geometric means or by electronic means. The former involves increasing the distance between the patient and the image intensifier tube; the latter involves collimating the beam automatically to fall only on a small central portion of the image intensifier input screen.
    - Both geometric and electronic magnification increase the patient dose in fluoroscopy, and require an increase in mA (to maintain the brightness of the television image), as described in section "Fluoroscopic Equipment Factors."
    - A dual-mode (25/17 cm) image intensifier tube will deliver 2.2 times ($25^2 \div 17^2$) more dose to the patient when operating in the 17 cm mode, or the magnification mode [1].

(a)

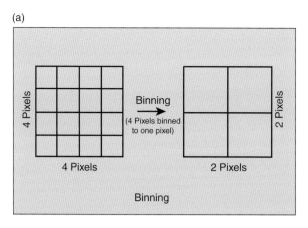

(b)

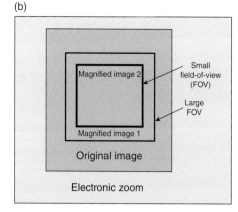

Figure 12.4 Electronic magnification in digital fluoroscopy includes binning (a) and electronic zooming (b).

- *Magnification in flat-panel digital (FPD) fluoroscopy systems.* There are two methods of magnification (Figure 12.4): *binning* (Figure 12.4a) and *electronic magnification* obtained through *electronic zooming* (Figure 12.4b). With electronic magnification, there is no increase in spatial resolution, and both original and magnified images have the same SNR. Furthermore, "binning has the disadvantage of less spatial resolution because the effective area of each image pixel is four times larger, and it has the advantage of lower data rates and less image mottle than ungrouped pixels" [11]. Electronic magnification uses collimation to select only the central portion of the FPD detector (similar with image intensifiers), as shown in Figure 12.4b. As Nickoloff [11] points out "when smaller FOVs are used, the data rate is lower, and binning is no longer required. Unlike image intensifier fluoroscopy systems, the spatial resolution of FPD fluoroscopy systems is the same for all FOVs – if no binning is employed. For those larger FOVs when binning is employed, the spatial resolution dramatically decreases to 50% of the value without binning. For FPD systems, there is a dramatic, discrete step change in spatial resolution between small and large FOVs."
- *LIH* is a technique used in fluoroscopy that refers to images that are stored digitally and displayed on the television monitor continuously without the need for fluoroscopy. Usually the last image is displayed on the monitor electronically for a period. Last-image-hold techniques can reduce patient dose by 50–80% [9].
- *Scattered radiation in fluoroscopy.* When conducting a fluoroscopic examination, both radiologists and technologists are exposed to scattered radiation by virtue of their presence in the room to assist the patient during the procedure. Important points to note in this situation are as follows:
  ○ The patient represents the main source of scattered radiation. The equipment is also a source of scattered radiation.
  ○ When the system is operated in what is referred to as the high dose rate mode, more scattered radiation is produced.
  ○ A higher level of scattered radiation reaches the fluoroscopist when the primary beam is off the patient's mid line, because there is less attenuation of the primary beam by the patient since it is closer to the operator.
  ○ The distribution of scattered radiation is higher when no protective curtain compared to when a protective curtain is used [1].

○ Occupational exposures in fluoroscopy can be reduced when lead protective aprons are worn. Technologists should always try to stand back from the table during beam-on times.
○ Personnel dosimeters must be worn at the level of the collar, outside the protective apron (in the United States) [1] and under the apron at the waist level (in Canada) [12] to record the dose from scattered radiation.

CT RADIATION DOSE FACTORS AND DOSE OPTIMIZATION CONSIDERATIONS

In Chapter 8, the essential physics and instrumentation of CT were described. In CT, the following topics relate to dose and include the dose distribution in the patient, dose metrics, factors affecting the dose, and dose optimization.

Dose distribution in the patient

The distribution of the dose in the patient in radiography is nonuniform, since the x-ray beam geometry is stationary (Figure 12.5a). This results in a dose distribution that is 100% at the surface of the patient and about 3% at the detector [8]. In CT, however, the dose distribution is more uniform at the surface of the patient and decreases toward the center because the scanning x-ray beam geometry rotates around the patient for 360° (Figure 12.5b). This significant difference requires additional CT dose descriptors or CT dose metrics.

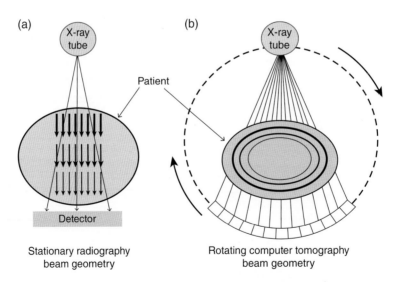

(a) Stationary radiography beam geometry

(b) Rotating computer tomography beam geometry

Figure 12.5   The distribution of the dose in the patient in radiography is nonuniform, since the x-ray beam geometry is stationary (a). This results in a dose distribution that is 100% at the surface of the patient and about 3% at the detector. In CT, however, the dose distribution is more uniform at the surface of the patient and decreases toward the center because the scanning x-ray beam geometry rotates around the patient for 360° (b).

CT dose metrics

There are at least four dose metrics used in CT dosimetry and they include the computed tomography dose index (CTDI), the dose length product (DLP), the size-specific dose estimate (SSDE), and the ED. The basics of these four metrics are described briefly here. For detailed descriptions, the reader should refer to Bushberg et al. [9]. In this chapter, only the first three will be described since the latter (ED) relates the radiation exposure to risk and is considered the best method available to estimate stochastic radiation risk [1, 6, 8, 9]. The following brief descriptions are significant to an understanding of the dose in CT:

* The typical dose distribution is a bell-shaped curve, as shown in Figure 12.6. The *dose distribution* is given by the function D(z), where D is the dose and z is the longitudinal axis of the patient (line drawn from head to toe). D(z) is extremely important to the CT dose because this is the dose distribution, or dose profile, that is measured.
* The *CTDI* is a standardized measure of the radiation output from a CT scanner and is used to compare the radiation output from different CT scanners.
* Specifically, the dose in the z-axis of the patient in the CT scanner is referred to as the $CTDI_{vol}$ for multi-slice CT (MSCT); it is expressed in milligray (mGy). The following algebraic expression is used to calculate the $CTDI_{vol}$:

$$CTDI_{vol} = \frac{CTDI_w}{pitch},$$

where the $CTDI_w$ is the weighted CTDI and it is used to account for the average dose in the x–y axis of the patient instead of the z-axis. For a pitch of 1, the $CTDI_{vol}$ is equal to the $CTDT_w$. The $CTDI_{vol}$ is not used to estimate the dose to the patient.

* The value of the $CTDI_{vol}$ is the same whether a technologist scans a 1- or 100-mm length of tissue. The *DLP* was introduced to provide a much more accurate representation of the dose for a defined length (L) of tissue in centimeters. The DLP provides a measure of the total dose for a CT, and can be calculated as follows:

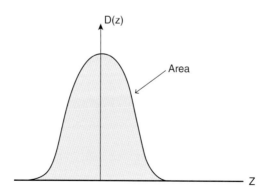

Figure 12.6 The typical dose distribution in CT is a bell-shaped curve. The dose distribution is given by the function D(z), where D is the dose and z is the longitudinal axis of the patient (line drawn from head to toe). D(z) is extremely important to the CT dose because this is the dose distribution, or dose profile, that is measured.

$$DLP = CTDI_{vol} \times L.$$

- The $CTDI_{vol}$ is the same regardless of the **size** of the patient; that is, the $CTDI_{vol}$ is the same for a large patient as it is for a small patient (keeping all scan parameters the same). Therefore, another metric is used to take into consideration the size of the patient.
- The *SSDE* is given by the formula:

$$SSDE_{16} = CTDI_{vol} \text{ (for a 16cm CTDI phantom)} \times \text{conversion factor } f \text{ (for the 16cm CTDI phantom)}$$

or

$$SSD_{32} = CTDI_{vol} \text{ (for a 32cm CTDI phantom)} \times \text{conversion factor } f \text{ (for the 32cm CTDI phantom)}.$$

Factors affecting the dose in CT

In this regard, Bushong [1] provides a mathematical expression which links the dose to a number of technical factors relating to image quality factors such as noise, contrast resolution, spatial resolution (defined by the pixel size and slice thickness) used in CT as follows:

$$Dose = k \cdot \frac{intensity \times beam\ energy}{noise^2 \times pixel\ size^3 \times slice\ thickness}$$

where k is a conversion factor, and the expression implies the following about dose and image quality:

- Reducing the noise in an image by a factor of 2 requires an increase in the dose by a factor of 4.
- Improving the spatial resolution (pixel size) by a factor of 2 requires an increase in the dose by a factor of 8.
- Decreasing the slice thickness by a factor of 2 requires an increase in the dose by a factor of 2 (keeping the noise constant).
- Decreasing both slice thickness and pixel size (spatial resolution) by a factor of 2 requires an increase in the dose by a factor of 16 ($2^3 \times 2 = 2 \times 2 \times 2 \times 2$).
- Increasing milliamperage and kilovolt peak increase patient dose proportionally. For example, a twofold increase in milliamperage increases the dose by a factor of 2. Additionally, doubling the dose requires an increase by the square of the kilovolt peak.

In addition to the factors listed above, several other factors influence the dose in CT and include the exposure technique factors, pitch, scan field-of-view, beam collimation, iterative reconstruction (IR) algorithms, gantry tilt, anatomical coverage, automatic exposure control (AEC), such as tube current modulation, whether a scanner is a single detector or a multidetector unit, overbeaming and overranging, patient centering, repeats, noise index, and improved detection efficiency. It is not within the scope of this Chapter to describe all of these factors; however, the following factors are worthy of a brief description:

- *Exposure technique factors*: The dose to the patient is directly proportional to the mAs and directly proportional to the square of the square of the kV change. Doubling the mAs will double the dose. Decreasing the kilovolt peak from 140 to 120 kV reduces the dose by

28–40% for a typical phantom [13], and further decreasing kV to 80 kV reduces the dose by approximately 65%. Precise adjustment of dose should not be obtained solely through manipulation of peak kilovoltage [13].

- *Pitch.* The dose is inversely proportional to the pitch, when all parameters remain constant. At 20 kV, 300 mA, 1 s, and 10 mm using a single-slice scanner (all factors held constant), the pitch for a body phantom has been shown to increase from 0.5 with a dose of 36 mGy, while a pitch of 2.0 decreases the CTDI_{vol} to 9 mGy. With the use of AEC, the tube current increases when the pitch is increased, and therefore it is not best practice to reduce exposure with MSCT scanners [13].

- *Collimation*: In CT, collimation defines the beam width and refers to the efficient use of the beam at the detector. For MSCT, the slice or section thickness (width) is defined by the number of detector elements grouped or binned together in each detector channel [1, 8, 9]. In general, as the collimation width increases (wider beam = thicker section), the dose decreases. As the section thickness decreases, the exposure must increase to maintain the same SNR as a thick section. A 2.5-mm section requires two times more exposure than a 5-mm section [13].

- *Section thickness*: The noise in CT is inversely proportional to the reconstructed or nominal section thickness. A section thickness of 2.5 mm will have increased noise (1.4 times more) than a 5-mm-thick section. Therefore, if a 2.5-mm-thin section is used in the examination, the technique factors (mAs and kV) must be increased to offset the increased noise associated with thinner sections [13].

- *AEC* is linked to the dose to the patient. For example, Toth et al. [14] reported that the ED in chest CT examinations was reduced by approximately 10%. Furthermore, longitudinal modulation accounts for two-thirds of dose reduction, and angular modulation accounts for the remaining one-third.

- *Image quality index:* An important feature of AEC systems is a preselected *image quality index*, also referred to as a *reference or target image quality index or noise index*. This index depends on several factors such as tube voltage, patient size, anatomic region, and the diagnostic task. The index is an operator-selectable parameter. The index is inversely proportional to the square root of the dose. When the noise index is reduced by 5%, the dose increases approximately 11%. If the noise index is increased by 5%, the dose is reduced by approximately 9% [15].

- *Overbeaming and Overranging*: *Overranging* refers to the use of additional rotations before and after the planned length of tissue so the first and last images can be reconstructed [16]. *Overbeaming* is the excess dose beyond the edge of the detector rows per rotation of a multi-section [16]. Figure 12.7 illustrates overbeaming and overranging. Both overranging and overbeaming increase radiation dose to the patient. Adaptive collimation is used in modern CT scanners to reduce patient dose at the beginning and end of scanning [17]. Christner et al. [18] demonstrated that dynamic collimation can reduce the dose by approximately 40%.

- *Iterative algorithms* (IR): The fundamental principles of a generalized IR algorithm were described in Chapter 8. Several studies have shown that IR algorithms can reduce the dose from 30 to 50% using IR [19]. A literature review showed that IR algorithms can reduce radiation dose and improve image quality in CT compared with filtered back-projection algorithms [20].

Dose optimization overview

The ALARA principle of the ICRP refers to *optimization* of the dose delivered to the patient during an examination. Specifically, it means maintaining a balance between the need for patient radiation protection (use of a dose that is ALARA) without compromising the quality of the images obtained. Optimization therefore deals with both radiation dose and image quality.

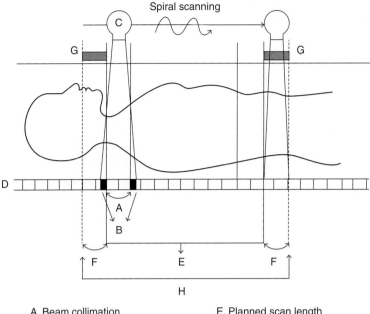

A. Beam collimation
B. Overbeaming
C. X-ray tube
D. Detector rows

E. Planned scan length
F. Overranging
G. Adaptive section collimation
H. Actual exposed length

Figure 12.7 The difference between overbeaming and overranging in CT. Adaptive or dynamic collimation also is illustrated. *Source*: Goo [16]. © 2012, The Korean Society of Radiology.

Research has continued to determine the best methods for lowering radiation dose in CT. These studies often are complex so they can follow precise scientific methods, including identifying the problem, performing a literature review, stating the goals regarding investigation of the problem, and designing a methodology to find a solution to the problem. Scientific methods also include data collection, analysis and interpretation of the data, and dissemination of the study findings.

In a special issue of the journal *Radiation Protection Dosimetry* dedicated to optimization strategies in medical imaging for fluoroscopy, radiography, mammography, and CT, several studies identified at least four important requirements for dose and image-quality optimization research [21]:

- Ensure patient safety.
- Determine the level of image quality required for a particular diagnostic task.
- Acquire images at various exposure levels from high to low and in such a manner that accurate diagnosis can still be made.
- Use reliable and valid methodologies for the dosimetry, image acquisition, and evaluation of image quality using human observers, keeping in mind the nature of the detection task.

References

1. Bushong, S. (2013). *Radiologic Science for Technologists*, 11e. St Louis, MO: Elsevier.
2. Kaza, R.K., Platt, J.F., Goodsitt, M.M. et al. (2014). Emerging techniques for dose optimization in abdominal CT. *Radiographics* 34: 4–17.
3. Fauber, T.L. and Dempsey, M.C. (2013). X-Ray field size and patient dosimetry. *Radiol. Technol.* 85 (2): 155–161.

4. Bomer, J., Wiersma-Deijl, L., and Holscher, H.C. (2013). Electronic collimation and radiation protection in paediatric digital radiography: revival of the silver lining. *Insight Imag.* 4: 723–727.

5. Joyce, M., McEntee, M., Brennan, P., and O''Leary, D. (2013). Reducing dose for digital cranial radiography: the increased source-to-the image-receptor distance approach. *J. Med. Imag. Radiat. Sci.* 44: 180–187.

6. Wolbarst, A.B., Capasso, P., and Wyant, A.R. (2013). *Medical Imaging: Essentials for Physicians*. Hoboken, NJ: Wiley.

7. Seeram, E. (2020). *Rad Techs Guide to Radiation Protection*. Hoboken, NJ: Wiley.

8. Seeram, E. and Brennan, P. (2017). *Radiation Protection in Diagnostic X-Ray Imaging*. Burlington, MA: Jones and Bartlett Learning, LLC.

9. Bushberg, J.T., Seibert, J.A., Leidholdt, E.M. Jr., and Boone, J.M. (2012). *The Essential Physics of Medical Imaging*, 3e. Philadelphia: Wolters Kluwer/Lippincott Williams & Wilkins.

10. Smith, D.L., Heldt, J.P., Richards, G.D. et al. (2013). Radiation exposure during continuous and pulsed fluoroscopy. *J. Endourol.* 27 (3): 384–388.

11. Nickoloff, E.L. (2011). Survey of modern fluoroscopy imaging: flat-panel detectors versus image intensifiers and more. *Radiographics* 31: 591–602.

12. Health Canada (2008). *Radiation Protection in Radiology-Large Facilities. Safety Code 35.* Ottawa: Ministry of Health.

13. Maldjian, P.D. and Goldman, A.R. (2013). Reducing radiation dose in body CT: primer on dose metrics and key CT technical parameters. *AJR Am. J. Roentgenol.* 200 (4): 741–774.

14. Toth, T., Ge, Z., and Daly, M.P. (2007). The influence of patient centering on CT dose and image noise. *Med. Phys.* 34 (7): 3093–3101.

15. Kanal, K.M., Stewart, B.K., Kolokythas, O., and Shuman, W.P. (2007). Impact of operator-selected image noise index and reconstruction slice thickness on patient radiation dose in 64-MDCT. *AJR Am. J. Roentgenol.* 189 (1): 219–225.

16. Goo, H.W. (2012). CT radiation dose optimization and estimation: an update for radiologists. *Korean J. Radiol.* 13 (1): 1–11.

17. Mattsson, S. and Söderberg, M. (2011). Radiation dose management in CT, SPECT/CT and PET/CT techniques. *Radiat. Prot. Dosim.* 147 (1–2): 13–21.

18. Christner, J.A., Zavaletta, V.A., Eusemann, C.D. et al. (2010). Dose reduction in helical CT: dynamically adjustable z-axis x-ray beam collimation. *AJR Am. J. Roentgenol.* 194 (1): W49–W55.

19. Beister, M., Kolditz, D., and Kalender, W.A. (2012). Iterative reconstruction methods in x ray CT. *Phys. Med.* 28 (2): 94–108.

20. Qiu, D. and Seeram, E. (2016). Does iterative reconstruction improve image quality and reduce dose in computed tomography? *Radiol. Open J.* 1 (2): 42–54.

21. Mattsson, S. (2005). Optimization strategies in medical x-ray imaging. *Radiat. Prot. Dosim.* 114 (1–3): 1–3.

13

Essential principles
of radiation protection

A Comprehensive Guide to Radiographic Sciences and Technology, First Edition. Euclid Seeram.
© 2021 John Wiley & Sons Ltd. Published 2021 by John Wiley & Sons Ltd.

INTRODUCTION

Radiation protection is an integral component of the curriculum for the education of medical imaging technologists, radiologists, and medical physicists working in radiology departments. Radiation Protection addresses the principles, techniques, and procedures used to protect patients, personnel, and members of the public. In diagnostic radiography, patients are the individuals who are exposed to the primary beam of x-rays from the x-ray tube needed to create the images used for the purpose of diagnosis; operators may by exposed to radiation scattered from the patient and/or the equipment. Members of the public, on the other hand, are those individuals who are working or waiting in close proximity to an x-ray room. Examples of these individuals include radiology support staff and family members of patients. Radiation protection includes a wide scope of topics ranging from biological factors, physical factors, technical factors, regulatory and guidance recommendations to procedural factors.

The purpose of this chapter is to outline these factors by focusing on the essential major concepts and principles that provide the necessary skills needed for competent operation of the equipment and application of the procedures that are the fundamental tools for optimization of the dose to patients.

WHY RADIATION PROTECTION?

The biological effects (harmful effects or health effects) of radiation exposure of humans have been studied extensively, and the results of these studies have been derived from a number of sources of data.

Categories of data from human exposure

There are a number of sources of data on human exposure to radiation [1] and they are as follows: early radiation workers such as radiologists and medical physicists who were exposed to high doses, workers in the radiation and nuclear industries, survivors of atomic bomb explosions at Hiroshima and Nagasaki, workers and local inhabitants exposed in the Three Mile Island and Chernobyl nuclear reactor accidents, and data on exposure of patients to high doses from medical radiation. The latter has been identified in the Biological Effects of Ionizing Radiation (BEIR Report VII) [2].

Radiation dose–risk models

Dose–Risk or Dose–Response Models were described in Chapter 11 on radiobiology. In summary, two Dose–Response models were identified: the *linear dose–response model without a threshold* (LNT model) and the linear dose–response model with a threshold. The *LNT model* implies that no amount of dose is considered safe, and that any dose, no matter how small, carries some degree of risk. The relationship shows that as the dose increases, the biologic response increases proportionately. The latter model proposes that no bioeffect is observed below a certain level of dose defined as the threshold dose, and that a biologic response occurs only when the threshold dose is reached, and that the response increases as the dose is increased [3–5].

Currently, radiation protection standards in medical imaging are based on the LNT model, since it is "a prudent basis for radiological protection makes summation of doses possible and drives optimization of protection. At high doses, risk is higher, and at low doses, risk is lower. Action should be commensurate with dose/risk. At low doses, action, if any, should be modest" [5].

Summary of biological effects

The risk models mentioned earlier are concerned with the biological effects (risks) as a consequence of radiation exposure (dose). In summary, biological effects (described in Chapter 11) have been placed into two categories: stochastic effects and deterministic effects.

- *Stochastic effects* are those effects for which the probability of occurrence increases as the dose increases, and for which there is no threshold dose. Any dose, no matter how small, carries the potential to cause biologic damage. There is no risk-free dose. Examples include cancer, leukemia, and genetic effects.
- *Deterministic effects* are those effects for which the severity of the effect increases with increasing dose and for which there is a threshold dose. Examples include radiation-induced skin burns, tissue damage, and organ dysfunction.

Radiation protection organizations/reports

There are a number of organizations, both internationally and nationally, that play significant roles in radiation protection in medicine, specifically in the development of radiation protection guides, recommendations, and control procedures on radiation safety. Examples of these organizations are:

- International Commission on Radiological Protection (ICRP).
- International Atomic Energy Agency (IAEA).
- National Council on radiation Protection and Measurements (NCRP) in the United States.
- Radiation Protection Bureau-Health Canada (RPB-HC) in Canada.
- Health Protection Agency (Formerly referred to as the National Radiological Protection Board (NRPB)) in the United Kingdom.

Examples of seminal reports of particular importance to radiologic technologists and radiologists include the following:

- ICRP Publication 93: Managing Patient Dose in Digital Radiology.
- ICRP Publication 103: The 2007 Recommendations of the ICRP.
- NCRP Report 172: Reference Levels and Achievable Doses in Medical and Dental Imaging – Recommendations for the United States.
- NCRP Report 160: Ionizing Radiation Exposure of the Population of the United States.
- Health Canada. Radiation Protection in Radiology – Large Facilities: Safety Code 35.
- NCRP Report 168: Radiation Dose Management for Fluoroscopically – Guided Interventional Medical Procedures.
- US Nuclear Regulatory Commission: Standards for Protection Against Radiation. US Code of Federal Regulations, 10 CFR 20.
- US Environmental Protection Agency. Federal Guidance Report 14: Radiation Protection Guidance for Diagnostic and Interventional X-Ray Procedures.

OBJECTIVES OF RADIATION PROTECTION

There are two fundamental goals of radiation protection and they are:

1. To *prevent the occurrence of deterministic effects* by ensuring that doses are kept below the threshold dose levels identified in the linear dose–response model with a threshold dose (D_T).
2. To minimize the induction of stochastic effects by adhering to a radiation protection philosophy which ensures optimization of the examination such that the best image quality is obtained using the minimum dose to the patient.

RADIATION PROTECTION PHILOSOPHY

The ICRP has identified and provides a *radiation protection framework* based on three philosophical pillars (Figure 13.1) on which the fundamental principles of radiation are founded [6, 7]. This framework is subscribed to by various national radiation protection organizations such as, for example, the NCRP and RPB-HC. These principles include justification, optimization, and application of dose limits. Each of these will be described briefly below.

Justification

The principle of justification calls for a good understanding of the benefits and risks of exposure to ionizing radiation. It implies that the net benefit should outweigh the risks. In this regard, the ICRP states that justification "should do more good than harm" for the patient [6]. Furthermore, the Food and Drug Administration (FDA) [8], in the United States, in promoting the ICRP principles on radiation protection, provides the following statement regarding justification:

"The imaging procedure should be judged to do more good than harm to the individual patient. Therefore, all examinations using ionizing radiation should be performed only when necessary to answer a medical question, help treat a disease, or guide a procedure. The clinical indication and patient medical history should be carefully considered before referring a patient for any examination."

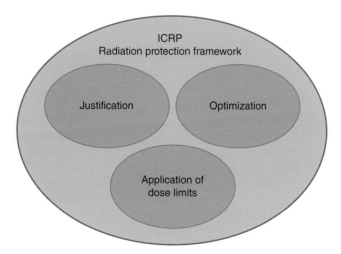

Figure 13.1 The three philosophical pillars of the ICRP on which the fundamental principles of radiation are founded. See text for further explanation.

An additionally noteworthy point about justification is one by Wolbarst et al. [9] who state that: "Justification provides an essential moral stance for the intelligence use of radiation."

Optimization

The ICRP principle of optimization refers to the use of techniques and procedures to reduce doses to patients and personnel. This principle is designed to ensure that the doses are kept **A**s **L**ow as **R**easonably **A**chievable (ALARA) without compromising the diagnostic quality of the image. The ICRP also uses the term Optimization of Radiation Protection (ORP). These two terms are synonymous.

There are several strategies for optimization of radiation protection, including the correct and accurate implementation of technical factors affecting the dose to the patient, such as the appropriate use of the correct exposure factors (kV and mAs) for example. These factors have been described in Chapter 12. Examples of other means of optimization include regulatory and guidance recommendations, diagnostic reference levels (DRLs), and gonadal shielding. These will be described subsequently.

An example of dose optimization in digital radiography is one by Seeram et al. [10], on the use of the exposure indicator (EI) to reduce the dose to the lumbar spine and pelvis. The results showed that optimized values of 16 mAs/EI = 136 for the anteroposterior (AP) pelvis and 32 mAs/EI = 139 for the AP lumbar spine did not compromise image quality. Selecting optimized mAs reduced dose by 36% compared with the vendor's recommended mAs (dose) values. Optimizing the mAs and associated EIs can be an effective dose management strategy.

Dose limits

The ICRP has established dose limits as another means of limiting the radiation risks. These limits have been issued for *occupationally exposed individuals* (those working with radiation, such as in medical imaging), and for *members of the public*, such as family members and others waiting for patients in the imaging department. There are no limits for patients.

Dose limits have been established to minimize the probability of stochastic effects based on the LNT model and are recommended by not only the ICRP but also by national radiation protection organizations such as the NCRP and RPB-HC. It should be noted that if these limits are exceeded, "appropriate measures should be put into place to minimize reoccurrence, and the exposed individual should be monitored for any adverse sequelae" [11]. Current (at the time of writing this chapter) dose limits from the ICRP [6], NCRP [12], and RPB-HC [13] are as follows:

- ICRP
    - *Occupational dose limit* is 20 mSv/year average over defined periods of five years.
    - Dose limits for the *eye lens, skin, and hands and feet* are 150, 500, and 500 mSv/year, respectively.
    - Dose limit for *members of the public* is 1 mSv annually, and are 15 and 50 mSv/year for the eye lens and skin, respectively.
- NCRP
    - Occupational dose limit is 50 mSv/year.
    - *Cumulative dose limit* is 10 mSv × age of the individual.
    - Dose limits for the *eye lens, skin, and hands and feet* are 150, 500, and 500 mSv/year, respectively.

    ◦ Dose limits for *students* (under the age of 18) in training is 1 mSv/year, while it is 15 mSv/year for lens of the eye, and 50 mSv/year for the skin, hands and feet, respectively. Additionally, occupational dose limits apply to students older than 18.

    ◦ Dose limits for *members of the public* is 1 mSv/year and are 15, 50, and 50 mSv for the eye lens, skin, hands and feet, respectively.

- RPB-HC
  ◦ Occupational dose limits and members of the public are the same as those of the ICRP.
  ◦ Dose limits for the *eye lens, skin, hands, and all other organs* are 15, 50, 50, and 50 mSv/year, respectively.
  ◦ For "technologists-in-training" and students in training, the annual dose limit is 1 mSv/year.
  ◦ For occupationally exposed women, once pregnancy has been declared, the fetus must be protected from x-ray exposure, for the remainder of the pregnancy. For women who are also occupationally exposed, an effective dose limit of 4 mSv must be applied, for the remainder of the pregnancy from all sources of radiation [13].

PERSONAL ACTIONS

The first triad of radiation protection is viewed as the ICRP's framework for radiation protection. The second triad shown in Figure 13.2 is referred to as *personal actions*, and includes the actions of time, shielding, and distance, which Bushong [3] has labeled as the "cardinal principles of radiation protection." These two triads provide the basis for radiation protection criteria and standards. Radiation dose to patients and personnel can be reduced as follows:

Time

The dose is directly proportional to the exposure time; if the time is doubled, the dose doubles proportionally. This simply means that ensure that the exposure time is kept as short as possible.

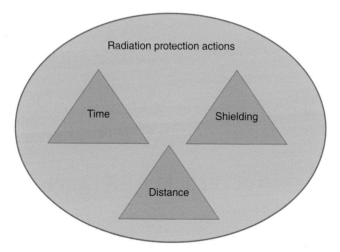

Figure 13.2 The second triad of radiation protection is referred to as personal actions, and includes the actions of time, shielding, and distance. See text for further explanation.

Furthermore, in radiographic imaging, short exposure times will minimize image blur due to patient motion. In fluoroscopic imaging, the beam-on time should be kept as short as possible to reduce exposure to the patient. Intermittent fluoroscopy will result in short beam-on times.

Shielding

Shielding implies the use of lead and or bismuth to shield patients' radiosensitive organs such as the gonads (gonadal shielding) and thyroid glands, for example, during an examination or wearing a lead apron in fluoroscopy and mobile radiography to protect technologists from unnecessary radiation scattered from the patient and equipment. *Gonadal shielding* has recently been a subject of debate as to its effectiveness, and will be discussed in a separate section in the chapter.

Shielding also includes x-ray room shielding which refers to shielding the walls of the x-ray rooms with lead to prevent radiation from exposing individuals outside the x-ray room (e.g. patients waiting for their examination in a waiting room that is in close proximity to x-ray rooms).

In wall shielding, the half-value layer (HVL) or the tenth-value layer (TVL) is used to estimate the amount of reduction of the radiation intensity by a protective barrier. While the HVL is the thickness of the shielding material that will reduce the intensity by one-half, the TVL is that thickness of material that will reduce the intensity by one-tenth of the original intensity. Lead or concrete can be used as wall shielding materials. At 80 kV, the HVL of lead is 0.19 mm, while it is 1.1 mm for concrete [3]. The basics of protective shielding will be described later in this chapter.

Distance

The intensity of radiation is inversely proportional to the square of the distance from the radiation source (x-ray tube, for example) As the distance increases, the radiation exposure decreases according to a physical law referred to as the *inverse square law*. The mathematical expression for this law is:

$$I \alpha \frac{1}{d^2},$$

where I = intensity of the radiation and d = distance. The expression is read as follows: the intensity of radiation is inversely proportional to the square of the distance. This means that a technologist engaged in mobile radiography should stand back the full length of the exposure cord. The regulatory guideline for the length of the exposure cord on a mobile x-ray unit must be 2 m (6 ft) long in the United States. The technologist should also wear a protective lead apron.

RADIATION QUANTITIES AND UNITS

The topic of radiation quantities and their associated units is important since exposure of humans to ionization radiation can arise from several sources. These sources will be reviewed briefly followed by a description of specific radiation quantities and their units of relevance to diagnostic radiology.

Sources of radiation exposure

These sources fall into two categories, namely, *natural environmental radiation* and *man-made radiation*. While the former consists of cosmic rays (particulate and electromagnetic radiation emitted by the sun and stars); terrestrial radiation (uranium deposits for example); internally deposited radionuclides [such as potassium 40 (^{40}K)]; and radon (radioactive gas as a result of the decay of uranium-238); the latter includes medical imaging and others such as nuclear power generation, research applications, industrial sources, and consumer devices [3].

An important consideration for technologists to remember is that of the natural environmental radiation, the largest source of population exposure in the United States arises from radon. Medical imaging includes modalities such as computed tomography (CT) scanning, radiography, interventional procedures, and nuclear medicine (NM) examinations. Of these, CT contributes the largest source of population exposures in the United States. While the average annual dose from natural environmental radiation is 3 mSv (2.0 mSv from radon, 0.3 mSv from cosmic, 0.3 mSv from terrestrial, and 0.4 mSv from internal), it is 3.2 mSv from medical imaging (1.5 mSv from CT, 0.7 mSv from NM, 0.6 from radiography, and 0.4 mSv from interventional) [14]. In 1990, as Bushong [3] points out the average patient dose from medical imaging was 0.6 mSv, compared with the 2008 reported average dose of 3.2 mSv from medical imaging, which is a "cause of considerable concern" [3].

In 2020, the Radiological Society of North America (RSNA) published a press release entitled "Medical Radiation Exposure Fell in the U.S. from 2006 to 2016." Mettler et al. [14] note the following in explaining this decrease:

- A key factor in the reduction was a substantial decrease in the number of nuclear medicine procedures, from 17 million in 2006 to 13.5 million in 2016.
- CT scans, a major driver of medical radiation exposure, increased from 67 million to 84 million scans over the 10-year period. However, the average individual effective dose from CT procedures dropped by 6%, thanks to several factors, according to study by coauthor Mahadevappa Mahesh, M.S., Ph.D., professor of radiology and cardiology at Johns Hopkins University School of Medicine in Baltimore.

Quantities and units

This chapter will address three radiation physical quantities of importance to radiation protection in diagnostic radiography. These include *exposure, absorbed dose*, and *effective dose*, since they are commonly used in practice and in studies reporting doses from radiology procedures. While exposure and absorbed dose refers to the radiation beam itself, the term effective dose relates to the biologic risk of the absorption of the radiation.

The units of these quantities are currently based on the *International System of Units* (SI units) which are now used throughout the world. Furthermore, in the United States, the NCRP as well as US scientific and medical societies have adopted SI units as early as in the 1990s [3].

- *Exposure* was the first radiation quantity and it relates to the task of the radiation to ionize air. The former unit (non-SI unit) was the *Roentgen* (R) (to honor Wilhelm Conrad Roentgen, who first discovered x-rays in 1895). The SI unit of exposure is the *coulomb per kilogram (C/kg)* where $1 R = 2.58 \times 10^{-4}$ C/kg: $1 C = 1.6 \times 10$ [15] electrons. Exposure follows the inverse square law (see above). This means that if the distance from the source of exposure (x-ray tube, for example) is increased by a factor of 2, then the exposure is decreased by a factor of 4. An important relationship applied to Nuclear Medicine (NM) is:

$$\text{Exposure} = \text{exposure rate} \times \text{time.}$$

- *Absorbed dose (D)* is the mean energy deposited by ionizing radiation to a medium (tissue) per unit mass, and represents the amount of energy absorbed by the medium. While the non-SI unit (old unit) is the *rad* (radiation absorbed dose), the SI unit is the *Gray* (Gy) where 1 Gy = 100 rads. Furthermore, 1 rad = 10 mGy (0.01 Gy). Additionally, 1 Gy = 1 Joule (J) per kilogram of absorbing material, and 1 J/kg = 1 Gy = 100 rads.
- *Effective dose (E)* is a quantity that relates exposure to biologic risks. Absorbed dose leads to excitation and ionization, physical processes leading to the production of free radicals. These free radicals subsequently result in biological damage. Historically, several quantities were used to quantify, such as dose equivalent (H) and equivalent dose (H_T). *Effective dose is the current quantity* (to be described later in this section). A brief description of the H and H_T follows:
  - *Dose equivalent (H)* represents a quantity that reflects the fact that different types of radiation have different efficiencies at producing biological damage. H = DQ, where D is the absorbed dose and Q is a quality factor addressing the effectiveness of the radiation to cause biological damage. For example, alpha particles have a higher *linear energy transfer* (LET) than diagnostic x-rays. 1 Gy of alpha particles can cause more damage that 1 Gy of diagnostic x-rays. LET is the efficiency of the radiation to cause excitation and ionization, and measures the rate at which energy is transferred to the living system. The unit of LET is the kilo-electron volt (kEV) per micrometer (μm) of length in soft tissue. As LET increases, biologic damage increases. For example, while the LET for diagnostic x-rays is about 3.0 keV/μm, it is 300 keV/μm for alpha particles.
  - In describing the efficiency with which the different types of radiation cause biologic damage in biologic systems, the term *Relative Biologic Effectiveness* (RBE) is thus used. Specifically, the RBE is a ratio of a standard (200–250 kV x-rays) radiation dose required to produce a given bioeffect to the test radiation dose needed to produce the same effect. The RBE for diagnostic x-rays is 1. As LET increases, RBE increases since high LET produces more ionization compared with low LET radiation.
  - The SI unit of H is the sievert (Sv) while the old (non-SI unit) was the rem (rad equivalent man). Sievert = Gray × Radiation Weighting Factor (W_R). 1 Sv = 100 rem; 1 mSv = 100 rem; 10 mSv = 1 rem. For the sake of simplicity, in radiology,

$$R = 1 \text{rad} = 1 \text{rem.}$$

In the SI units:

$$2.58 \times 10^{-4} \, \text{C} / \text{kg} = 0.01 \text{Gy} = 0.01 \text{Sv.}$$

  - As noted earlier, bioeffects not only depend on D but also on the type and energy of the radiation. For example, W_R for x-rays and gamma rays is 1, while it is 5 for high-energy protons, and 20 for alpha particles and fission fragments.
  - *Equivalent dose* (H_T) was introduced by the ICRP in 1990, in its revised recommendations and H was replaced by (H_T). While H is the weighted absorbed dose at a point, H_T is the weighted absorbed dose in tissues or organs.

$$H_T = \Sigma W_R D_{TR.}$$

- This expression states that the equivalent dose is equal to the sum of the weighted absorbed doses. D_{TR} is the absorbed dose averaged over the tissue or organ T, for the type of radiation R.
- *Effective dose* (E) takes into consideration the fact that different tissues have different radio-sensitivities [3] and is therefore weighted for the type of tissue (organ). E is used to quantify the different risks from partial body exposure compared with risks from an equivalent whole-body dose. E is calculated as follows:

$$E = \Sigma W_T H_T,$$

where W_T is the tissue weighting factor.
- The SI unit for E is the sievert (Sv).
- If the E for an upper gastrointestinal tract (UGT) examination is 2.45 mSv, then this value means that the risk from an UGT examination is equivalent to the risk of an exposure dose of 2.45 mSv to the whole body.
- The W_T for the gonads, active bone marrow, breast, and thyroid, for example, are 0.20, 0.12, 0.05, and 0.05, respectively.

PERSONNEL DOSIMETRY

Personnel dosimetry refers to the measurement and monitoring of the amount of radiation exposure received by occupationally exposed individuals. In medical imaging, a number of devices are used, including, optically stimulated luminescent dosimeter, thermoluminescent dosimeter (TLD), film dosimeter, and ionization chamber dosimeter. Only the first two will be reviewed briefly (since they are more commonplace) as follows:

- *Optically stimulated luminescence dosimetry* (OSLD). This is one of the most current methods used today known for its sensitivity and its detection of very small doses, compared to TLD. It was introduced in the late 1990s for recording personnel doses. The OSLD is based on the physical principle of optically stimulated luminescence (OSL) of the radiation detector. The detector is made of *carbon-doped aluminum oxide* (Al_2O_3 : C). There are three major steps in the manner the dosimeter is used, as shown in Figure 13.3, namely, exposure of the dosimeter, readout, and analysis. First, the OSLD detector is exposed to x-rays which causes electrons in the ground state (lower energy level) to move to an excited state (higher energy level) where they are trapped until they are optically stimulated by a laser light. Such laser stimulation causes the trapped electrons to fall back into their ground state, resulting in visible light emission. In the third step, this light is captured by a photodiode and the analysis provides a readout of the dose received by the dosimeter. The light intensity is

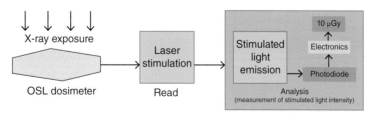

Figure 13.3 The use of the OSL dosimeter involves at least three major steps, namely, exposure of the dosimeter, readout, and analysis. See text for further explanation.

directly proportional to the amount of radiation received by the Al_2O_3 : C. The minimum dose that can be detected by the OLSD is $10\,\mu Gy$. The detection of such low doses is one of the major advantages of the OSLD over the TLD dosimeter [3].

- *Thermoluminescent dosimetry.* Thermoluminescent dosimetry uses the TLD. TLDs have been used as personnel dosimeters for years in radiology departments (and perhaps still being used today). The TLD is based on the physical principle of thermoluminescence, that is, the emission of light by a crystal after it has been exposed to x-rays. The most widely used crystal is *lithium fluoride* (LiF) although other crystals such as lithium borate, calcium fluoride, and calcium sulfate have been used as well [3]. There are basically three major steps involved when using the TLD: exposure to x-rays, heating, and subsequent analysis (Figure 13.4) and described in detail by Bushong [3]. First, exposure to x-rays causes the electrons in the ground state (lower energy state) to be raised and trapped in a higher energy state (excited state). These trapped electrons when heated to a specific degree, return to their original ground state emitting light in the process. Finally, the emitted light is captured by a photomultiplier tube (PMT) and analyzed to provide a dose reading. The light intensity is proportional to the dose received by the TLD. The TLD "can measure doses as low as $50\,\mu Gy$ (5 rad) with modest accuracy, and at doses exceeding $100\,\mu Gy$ (10 rad), its accuracy is better that 5%" [3].

- *Wearing the personnel dosimeter.* Personnel in medical imaging (radiography, fluoroscopy, and CT) must wear dosimeters to record their occupational exposures, in millisieverts.
  - Most radiation protection organizations recommend that in radiography, dosimeters be worn at the level of waist, at the level of the collar in the upper chest region, or on the anterior surface of the individual.
  - In fluoroscopy, when a protective apron must be worn, the NCRP [16] states that:
  When an apron is worn, a decision must be made as to whether to wear one or more than one dosimeter. If only one is worn, and it is worn under the apron, it can represent the dose to most internal organs, but it may underestimate the dose to the head and neck (including the thyroid gland). If only one is worn and it is worn at the collar, it may represent the dose to the organs contained in the head and neck, but it may overestimate the dose to the organs in the trunk of the body.
  - In Canada, the radiation protection Safety Code SC 35 [13] states that in fluoroscopy, the dosimeter must be worn under the apron; and when the radiation levels are considered to be high, additional dosimeters should be worn on the extremities.

An important point about personnel dosimeters is that "we assume the occupational dose to be 10% of the monitor dose. Assuming the effective dose of 10% of the occupational monitor dose is conservative. In actual fact, it is something less that 10%" [3]

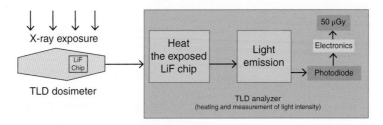

Figure 13.4   Three major steps involved when using the TLD: exposure to x-rays, heating, and subsequent analysis. See text for further explanation.

OPTIMIZATION OF RADIATION PROTECTION

The *optimization of radiation protection* refers to various measures that can be used to ensure that patients and personnel received doses according to the ALARA philosophy. Such measures for dose management, for example, include the following (not in any order): regulatory and guidance recommendations, the use of DRLs, gonadal shielding, x-ray protective shielding, and campaigns to promote radiation awareness and safety. Each of these will be examined briefly as follows:

Regulatory and guidance recommendations

These refer specifically to radiation protection reports, prepared by experts in the field of radiation protection, which focus on the mandatory requirements of the design and performance of imaging equipment, and offer regulations (*regulatory agencies*), as well as advisory recommendations on the safe use of the equipment and procedures used to image patients and to protect personnel working in diagnostic radiology departments, that come from *advisory bodies*. It is important for students, practitioners, and teaching staff refer to the reports relevant to their respective countries. For example, the US Food and Drug Administration (FDA) have jurisdiction over manufacturers who must confirm to various regulations on the design and performance aspects of equipment for use in the United States. Examples of an international advisory body is the ICRP. The advisory body in the United States and Canada are the NCRP and Health Canada-Radiation Protection Bureau.

Guidance recommendations have been developed for equipment design and performance, personnel practices, and quality assurance/quality control (QA/QC). It is not within the scope of this chapter to outline the details of these recommendations; however, only a few major ones will be highlighted to stress the importance of relevance to the optimization of radiation protection that technologists must pay careful attention to when imaging patients and practicing their craft. Furthermore, recommendations use the terms "shall" and "should" defined below in NCRP Reports, for example.

- *Definitions of "shall" and "should":* The exact meanings of each of these in NCRP Report No. 102 are: "Shall" and "shall not" are used to indicate that adherence to recommendations is necessary to meet current radiation protection standards. "Should" and "should not" are used to indicate a prudent practice to which exceptions may be occasionally made in appropriate circumstances [17]. In Canada, RPB-HC [13] defines the terms "must" and "should" as: "must, indicates a requirement that is essential to meet currently accepted standards of protection, while should indicates an advisory recommendation that is highly desirable and is to be implemented where practicable."
- *Equipment design and performance recommendations: radiography.* There are numerous recommendations for radiography; however, only a few will be highlighted here. These include filtration, collimation and beam alignment, source-to-skin distance (SSD), source-to-image receptor (SID), and the exposure switch, which are significant parameters relating to dose optimization.
  - *Filtration* removes the low-energy radiation from the heterogeneous beam from the x-ray tube, and in this manner. Filtration includes inherent plus added and together refers to *total filtration*. Filtration protects the patient from unnecessary radiation. All radiographic equipment must have added filtration in the x-ray beam. The material used in diagnostic x-ray imaging is aluminum (Al) and the thickness depends on the magnitude of the kV used. The minimum total filtration are as follows:
  1. If the operating kV is above 70, then the minimum total filtration shall be 2.5 mm aluminum equivalent.

2. If the operating kV is between 50 and 70, then the minimum total filtration shall be 1.5 mm aluminum equivalent.

3. If the operating kV is below 50, then the minimum total filtration shall be 0.5 mm aluminum equivalent.

    ○ *Collimation and beam alignment.* The recommendation requires that the x-ray field and the light beam must be aligned to within 2% of the SID distance.

    ○ *SID and SSD.* The SID must be accurate to within 2% of the SID used for the examination. Furthermore, the SID should not be less that 100 cm (40 in.) for table top examinations. The SSD (which determines the concentration of photons per unit area on the surface of the patient – shorter SSD results in more dose) shall not be less than 30 cm (12 in.) and should not be less than 38 cm (15 in.).

    ○ *Exposure switch.* The exposure switch on radiographic units shall be of the "dead man" type. This means that pressure must be applied to the switch for the exposure to occur. Since the technologist is in direct contact with this switch, recommendations require that for *fixed radiographic equipment*, the exposure switch must be located on the control panel to ensure that the operator remains in the control booth (protective booth) during the exposure. For mobile radiographic units, the exposure switch shall be attached to a long cord that allows the operator to stand at least 2 m (6 ft) from the patient and the unit. In Canada, the cord length must be 3 m long.

- *Equipment design and performance recommendations: fluoroscopy.* As noted for radiography, there are several recommendations for fluoroscopy, however, only the following will be highlighted: filtration, collimation, SSD, exposure switch, cumulative timer, protective curtain, and accessory protective clothing.

    ○ *Filtration.* In fluoroscopy, filtration is mandatory since high kVs are generally used and exposure times (beam-on times) are longer than in radiography. The minimum total filtration must be at least 2.5 mm aluminum equivalent.

    ○ *Collimation.* The NCRP [17] recommends that the collimator should be coupled and centered to the image receptor and should be confined to the image receptor at any SID.

    ○ *SID.* The SID in fluoroscopy shall not be less than 38 cm (15 in.) for fixed fluoroscopic systems and shall not be less than 30 cm (12 in.) for mobile fluoroscopic systems.

    ○ *Exposure switch.* This switch must be of the "dead man" type. Furthermore, the "foot switch" must be of the "dead man" type as well.

    ○ *Cumulative timer.* This timer is intended to record the length of time the beam is on for the entire examination. It should provide the operator with an audible tone or visual signal when five minutes of beam-on time have elapsed. Additionally, the signal should last for 15 seconds at which time it must be reset to continue fluoroscopy.

    ○ *Protective curtain.* This is a lead curtain or drape that hangs from the unit in such a manner that it protects the operator from scattered radiation from the patient during the examination. The dimensions should not be less than 45.7 cm × 45.7 cm (18 in. × 18 in.), and should have at least 0.25 mm lead-equivalent thickness.

    ○ *Protective clothing.* This refers to lead aprons, thyroid shields, and lead gloves worn by the operator. While aprons shall have at least 0.5 mm of lead-equivalent thickness, thyroid shields shall have at least 0.5 mm lead-equivalent thickness, and protective gloves shall have at least 0.5 mm lead-equivalent thickness.

Diagnostic reference levels (DRLs)

DRLs are a useful tool for optimization of patient radiation protection. Dose limits have been established for occupationally exposed individuals, and members of the public. The notion of DRLs was introduced by the ICRP in 1990, and is now being used by organizations, including the ICRP, NCRP, and HC-RPB in SC-35. A comprehensive explanation of the DRL is provided by Seeram and Brennan [11]; however, Seeram [18] summarizes the major features of the DRL as follows:

- "The DRL is an advisory, not a regulatory, measure. It is not related to dose limits established for radiation workers and members of the public.
- The DRL is intended to identify high levels of radiation dose to patients.
- The DRL applies to common examinations and specific equipment.
- Dose quantities and techniques should be easy to measure (e.g. the entrance skin exposure).
- The DRL selection is established by professional organizations, using a percentile point on the observed distribution for patients, and specific to a country or region. One pragmatic method is to use what has been referred to as a diagnostic reference range. While the upper level of the range is established at 75th percentile, the lower level is set at 25th percentile of the computed patient dose.
- Below a 25th percentile level, image quality may be compromised; above the 75th percentile may indicate excessive dose.
- For actual DRL values for various imaging examinations, the reader should consult their respective national radiation protection organizations."

The American College of Radiology (ACR), the American Association of Physicists in Medicine (AAPM), and the Society for Pediatric Radiology (SPR) have issued the following DRLs: for example, for the adult PA chest (23 cm patient thickness with grid), AP abdomen (22 cm patient thickness), and the AP lumbosacral spine (22 cm patient thickness) to be 0.15, 3.4, and 4.2 mGy, respectively [19].

Gonadal shielding: past considerations

For the past several decades, "patient shielding was-and is-justified as a matter of protection from hereditary risks, not as an overall reduction in stochastic risk. Of importance, 42 years later, no hereditary effects from radiation have ever been observed in humans" [15]. In the past months, however, there has been a debate about the use of gonadal shielding in medical imaging, as to whether shielding increases the radiation dose to the patient. With this notion in mind, several papers appeared in the literature addressing the advantages and disadvantages of gonadal shielding. The current state of gonadal shielding will be reviewed briefly in a separate section of this chapter. Previous major ideas for gonadal shielding were as follows:

- The correct use of a 1 mm lead-equivalent shield will reduce the gonadal dose by about 50% for females and about 90–95% for males [20].
- The thickness of the lead shield used for gonadal shielding must be at least 0.5 mm lead-equivalent [11].
- In 2012, the major objective of a study about gonadal shielding [21] was to re-evaluate shielding the gonads in children with respect to reducing the radiation risk, and loss of diagnostic information, in an effort to address the ICRP's optimization principle. The results of this study showed that "with modern optimized x-ray systems, the reduction of the detriment adjusted risk by gonadal shielding is negligibly small. Given the potential consequences of loss of diagnostic information, of retakes, and shielding of automatic exposure chambers, gonadal shielding might better be discontinued." The current status of gonadal shielding will be reviewed briefly in the next section of this chapter.

X-ray room shielding

Shielding x-ray rooms is intended to protect personnel and members of the public from unnecessary radiation. Lead in most cases is used (concrete may also be used for this purpose). The thickness of the lead depends on whether the wall is exposed by the primary beam (primary protective barriers) or to scattered radiation (secondary protective barrier). Lead may not be used for shielding secondary barriers since its four layers of thickness may be too thin (<0.4 mm). Therefore, lead acrylic gypsum brand of glass may be used (⅝ in. gypsum board with ½ in. plate glass will offer adequate protection). Furthermore, the control booth is considered a secondary protective barrier and is subject to the same lead thickness criterion for secondary barriers (the primary beam must never be directed toward the control booth). As described by Seeram [18], several factors that affect the thickness of protective barriers in radiology, and include the exposure rates for controlled and uncontrolled areas occupied by individuals, are the distance between the radiation source and the barrier, workload, occupancy factor, use factor (illustrated in Figure 13.5), and the kV used for examinations. The following descriptions are noteworthy [18]:

- A *controlled area* is an area in which an individual is occupationally exposed and includes radiology personnel and patients as well. Barriers for controlled areas must minimize the exposure rate to less than 1 mSv\week (100 mrem/wk).
- An *uncontrolled area* is the one occupied by any individual. Barriers for uncontrolled areas must reduce the exposure rate to that of members of the public, that is, 1 mSv/yr. (100 mrem/yr).
- Barriers for uncontrolled areas contain more lead than do barriers for controlled areas.
- The *workload* refers to the number of examinations performed per week, expressed as milli-ampere-minutes per week (mA-min/wk).
- The *occupancy factor* refers to the time that the area is occupied, expressed as a fraction of the work week. Levels of occupancy can be full (1), partial (1/4), and occasional (1/16) occupancy.

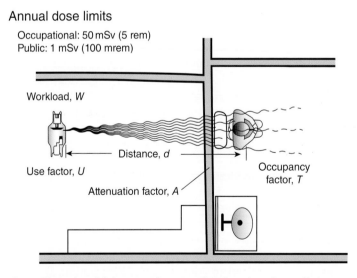

Figure 13.5 Factors that affect the thickness of protective barriers in radiology, and include the exposure rates for controlled and uncontrolled areas occupied by individuals, the distance between the radiation source and the barrier, workload, occupancy factor, and use factor. *Source*: Wolbarst [22]. © 2005, Medical Physics Pub.

- The *use factor* is the fraction of time during which the primary beam is on and aimed at the barrier. Use factors are provided for levels of full use (1), partial use (1/4), and occasional use (1/16).
- The maximum and average kV must also be known for calculating barrier thickness. The barrier thickness can be determined by referring to precalculated shielding requirement tables or by performing a calculation using the data for the various factors previously identified.

A detailed description of x-ray room shielding is provided by Seeram and Brennan [11].

CURRENT STATE OF GONADAL SHIELDING

Several authors [15, 21, 23–25] have discussed the justification for the discontinuation of the use of gonadal shielding in medical imaging. In 2019, the AAPM [26] issued a policy statement on the effectiveness of gonadal shielding as follows:

Patient gonadal and fetal shielding during X-ray based diagnostic imaging should be discontinued as routine practice. Patient shielding may jeopardize the benefits of undergoing radiological imaging. Use of these shields during X-ray based diagnostic imaging may obscure anatomic information or interfere with the automatic exposure control of the imaging system. These effects can compromise the diagnostic efficacy of the exam, or actually result in an increase in the patient's radiation dose. Because of these risks and the minimal to nonexistent benefit associated with fetal and gonadal shielding, AAPM recommends that the use of such shielding should be discontinued [26].

This position statement has received support and endorsement from several groups including the ACR, Australasian College of Physical Scientists and Engineers in Medicine (ACPSEM), Canadian Association of Radiologists (CAR), Canadian Organization of Medical Physicists (COMP), Health Physics Society (HPS) Image Gently, and the Radiological Society of North America (RSNA).

References

1. Hendee, W.R. and O'Connor, M.K. (2013). Radiation risks of medical imaging: separating fact from factasy. *Radiology* 204 (2): 312–320.
2. National Research Council (2006). *Health Effects from Exposure to Low Levels of Ionizing Radiation: BEIR Phase 2: Committee to Assess Health Risks from Exposure to Low Levels of Ionizing Radiation*. Washington, DC: National Academies Press.
3. Bushong, S. (2017). *Radiologic Science for Technologists*, 11e. Elsevier: St Louis, MO.
4. Tran, L. and Seeram, E. (2017). Current perspectives on the use of the linear non-threshold (LNT) in radiation protection. *International Journal of Radiology and Medical Imaging* 3: 123–128.
5. Clement, C. (2020). ICRP views on radiation risk at low doses through the lens of Fukushima. *Health Physics* 118 (3): 311–316.
6. ICRP (2007). ICRP publication no. 103: the 2007 recommendations of the international commission on radiological protection. *Annals of the ICRP* 37 (2–4): 1–332.
7. ICRP (2007). ICRP publication no. 105: radiation protection in medicine. International Commission on Radiological Protection. *Annals of the ICRP* 37 (6): 1–63.
8. FDA (2020). White paper: initiative to reduce unnecessary radiation exposure from medical imaging. https://www.fda.gov/radiation-emitting-products/initiative-reduce-unnecessary-radiation-exposure-medical-imaging/white-paper-initiative-reduce-unnecessary-radiation-exposure-medical-imaging (accessed July 2020).

9. Wolbarst, A.B., Capasso, P., and Wyant, A.R. (2013). *Medical Imaging: Essentials for Physicians*. Hoboken, NJ: Wiley.

10. Seeram, E., Davidson, R., Bushong, S., and Swan, H. (2016). Optimization of the exposure indicator of a CR system as a radiation dose management strategy. *Radiologic Technology* 87: 380–391.

11. Seeram, E. and Brennan, P. (2017). *Radiation Protection in Diagnostic X-Ray Imaging*. Burlington, MA: Jones and Bartlett learning.

12. NCRP (1993). Limitation of Exposure to Ionizing Radiation. Bethesda, MD. *Report No 116*.

13. Health Canada (2008). *Radiation Protection in Radiology – Large Facilities: Safety Code 35*. Ottawa: Ministry of Health.

14. Mettler, F.A. Jr., Thomadsen, B.R., Bhargavan, M. et al. (2008). Medical radiation exposure in the US in 2006: preliminary results. *Health Physics* 95 (5): 502–507.

15. Marsh, R.M. and Silosky, M. (2019). Patient shielding in diagnostic imaging: discontinuing a legacy practice. *AJR* 212: 755–757.

16. NCRP (1989). Exposure of the US Population from Occupational Radiation. Bethesda, MD. *NCRP Report No 101*.

17. NCRP (2015). Medical X-Ray, Electron Beam, and Gamma-Ray Protection for Energies up to 50 MeV (Equipment Design, Performance and Use. Bethesda, MD. *NCRP Report 102*.

18. Seeram, E. (2020). *Rad Tech's Guide to Radiation Protection*, 2e. Oxford: Wiley.

19. American College of Radiology ACR-AAPM-SPR (2018). Practice parameter for diagnostic reference levels and achievable doses in medical x-ray imaging. https://www.acr.org/–/media/ACR/Files/Practice-Parameters/Diag-Ref-Levels.pdf (accessed 30 August 2020).

20. Statkiewicz-Sherer, M.A., Visconti, P.J., Ritenour, E.R., and Haynes, K. (2012). *Radiation Protection in Medical Radiography*, 7e. Mosby: St Louis, MO.

21. Frantzen, M., Robben, S., Postma, A.A. et al. (2012). Gonadal shielding in paediatric pelvic radiography: disadvantages prevail over benefit. *Insights Imaging* 3: 23–32.

22. Wolbarst, A.B. (2005). *Physics of Radiology*, 2nde. Medical Physics Pub Corp.

23. Jeukens, C.R., Kütterer, G., Kicken, P.J. et al. (2020). Gonad shielding in pelvic radiography: modern optimised X-ray systems might allow its discontinuation. *Insights into Imaging* 11: 15.

24. GE Healthcare (2020). The shielding controversy in radiology. https://www.gehealthcare.com/long-article/the-shielding-controversy-in-radiology (accessed 20 August 2020).

25. Marsh, R.M. (2020). Patient shielding in 2020. *Journal of the American College of Radiology* 17 (9): 1183–1185.

26. AAPM (2019). AAPM position statement on the use of patient gonadal and fetal shielding. https://www.aapm.org/org/policies/details.asp?id=468&type=PP (accessed 30 August 2020).

Index